What Covid-19 Must Teach Us

What Covid-19 Must Teach Us

Meeting viruses with fear or informed common sense?

Dr. Thomas Hardtmuth

First in the Covid Perspectives series

A valuable reference work for evaluating Covid-19 responses as well as for any future health crises

InterActions

Stroud, UK

First published in German as
Gesunder Menschenverstand oder Angst
im Umgang mit COVID-19,
a section in
Corona und das Rätsel der Immunität,
Akanthos Akademie Edition

Original text revised and updated
by the author for this new English edition.
Translation by
Bernard Jarman

Published in the UK by
InterActions 2021
Second revised edition March 2022

www.interactions360.org
contact@interactions360.org

ISBN 978-0-9528364-7-6

Layout and Editing: InterActions
Printed in the UK
by ImprintDigital.com

Important note:
All medical descriptions in this text are for information,
and readers must decide for themselves what individual actions
they take following on from them. It is not intended as a substitute
for direct medical advice in the case of illness.

Contents

Foreword

The corona pandemic is keeping the world on tenterhooks. We all know that there will be no return to the old normal. But it seems all the more urgent to learn from the crisis. How could it come to this? What is the role of viruses in nature's household? How is our treatment of animals, indeed of the entire ecosystem, related to the pandemic, i.e. to our health? But the central question is: how does the immune system work? And above all: what does fear do to the immune system?

Fear and uncertainty have spread across all generations to a frightening extent. Overcoming fear requires a realistic assessment of the actual danger, and common sense. Thomas Hardtmuth addresses all these questions in this book. In addition to his work as a doctor, he has for years been dealing specifically with the nature of viruses, and has described their role in the household of nature in various publications.

For the idea that vaccination will solve the problem falls short of the mark. We are not only dealing with a virus but also with the susceptibility of the organism, i.e. with the question of what strengthens or weakens the human immune system. It is Thomas Hardtmuth's great concern to reveal the complex interrelationships that are causally connected to the pandemic. He wants to contribute to an objective and open discussion that takes all relevant dimensions into account and thus arrive at a holistic picture of the corona pandemic – which is urgently needed for the future of medicine and health. Such a genuine and fair discussion is – according to Hardtmuth – 'the basis of any healthy human culture'.

In this sense, I hope that the book will attract many interested readers who are committed to such a culture.

Michaela Glöckler, MD

April 2021

Preface to this edition

Viruses cannot be fought and certainly not eradicated. They are present everywhere in unbelievably large numbers. All the organisms on this earth are colonised by countless viruses of different kinds which are continually mutating, forming and disappearing again. Viruses can be seen as the dynamic building blocks of life that have existed since evolution began and have played a decisive role in our genetic development and the diversity of species in nature. Without viruses there could be no life on earth.

For more than two years a global battle has been raging against one of these millions of viruses in the belief that it poses a threat to the whole of mankind. The world community has been subject to a never-ending diet of media-induced fear scenarios, calls to engage in the fight against this invisible enemy, suffer considerable sacrifices and accept numerous repressive measures until humanity has been rescued from this danger and fear by a vaccine.

Is this fear justified? Is the narrative correct? There was widespread resistance in all parts of society from the very beginning and particularly in the field of science. After all anyone familiar with the subject matter will very quickly realise that something is not right – especially when all critical voices and the many reasonable questions were being categorically excluded or ignored. The unequivocal political message is that in this highly dangerous situation no one should question those with the sole responsibility for delivering us from this crisis. Where the legitimacy for the suspension of all democratic ground rules came from in this self-declared pandemic management is not said. It is the lack of transparency, the clearly alarmist manipulation of data and the apparent lack of any alternative to the rigorous imposition of a global vaccination campaign that has awakened mistrust in the population. 'Alternative thinkers' only arise when 'mainstream thinkers' (whatever these terms mean) become suspect, when their authoritarian power is used to suppress different opinions. In writing this book the aim has been to offer a contribution towards an open and differentiated dialogue.

In this new edition numerous points have been brought up to date and extended.

How do social, cultural and psychological factors affect our immune functions? Do vaccines make sense, what risks are connected with them, and why should children not be vaccinated against Covid?

Research into the microbiome is currently revolutionising our medical thinking and – especially in these corona times – offers an opportunity for developing an entirely new, integrated understanding of micro-organisms and viruses.

The economic motives, strategies and vast profits made in connection with the pandemic are also presented in detail.

With the rapidly advancing digital networks the possibilities for manipulating opinion and their wide reach has grown enormously. That is why there is an additional detailed chapter on aspects of media psychology and the misuse of power with refined propaganda techniques.

February 2022

Overview

The corona crisis provokes fear and confusion in large sections of the population. Most people find the scientific pronouncements about the pandemic hard to follow and often so contradictory that forming an opinion scarcely seems possible while any vestige of common sense is in danger of drowning in a sea of media panic. An ongoing state of confusion, fear and disorientation can be highly damaging not only to our health but also to the psycho-sociological climate and cohesion of society.

A worrying degree of uniformity permeates the handling of the corona crisis by the media. Lively debate which should be an essential part of every modern and enlightened, democratic society, is missing. There is growing scepticism and public unease about a creeping health dictatorship similar to that described ten years ago by Juli Zeh in her novel *Corpus delicti*. It is the absence of public debate and the ignoring of critical viewpoints that creates a fertile soil for scepticism, radicalisation and conspiratorial beliefs.

Our understanding of viruses and their significance for human beings and nature has also changed fundamentally over the last two decades, but very little of this is known despite their having dominated the headlines for months.[1] Viruses are the oldest, commonest and most widespread entities to have emerged during the course of evolution. Their role in illness cannot be understood unless we grasp the fact that viruses are essentially the primal building blocks of life. Without understanding them and knowing their significance for both human health and the natural world, their role in illness cannot be understood.

The following text will therefore attempt to clarify some of the essential facts underlying the current pandemic which are being misrepresented in the mainstream media with worrying consequences.

The importance of viruses

Viruses can be understood as 'elementary particles' within the greater web of life. To consider them out of context as the sole cause of illness no longer reflects current scientific thinking and is the consequence of an out-of-date bio-mechanistic understanding of nature and the human being which relies on an isolated chain of causes but cannot grasp the systemic relationships which are so vital for understanding micro-organisms. So long as we continue to see viruses as the enemy and misuse them to instil fear, the real and many-sided causes of global infections will be overlooked. The crisis offers a real learning opportunity.

Viruses are the most widespread entities found in nature. There are some 10^{31} viruses on earth; they make up a major part of the total biomass. For comparison: the number of grains of sand on earth is estimated at about 10^{20}. We would have to multiply this number by 100 billion to arrive at the number of viruses. Lining up all the viruses in the sea would result in a distance of 10 million light years.[2]

Viruses are largely made up of genetic material contained in a capsid. Some viruses also have an additional envelope, but this comes from a host cell – that is from another organism. The simplest and earliest forms of virus are the so-called virions which consist of a ring-shaped strand of RNA. They were present when life first began to develop, a concept paraphrased by 'the RNA world' or 'virus first' hypothesis. The development of physical life began with the RNA, which is why the genetic code applies universally to all forms of life – micro-organisms, plants, animals and humans all have the same basic structure of genetic code which may be imagined as a text. In the case of RNA it consists of 4 nucleobases analogous to the letters: Adenin (A), Cytosin (C), Guanin (G) and Uracil (U). With DNA the Uracil is replaced by Thymin 21 (T). The DNA – and RNA viruses – may contain either single or double stranded DNA or RNA, with the double stranded always having the corresponding base pairs – Adenin-Thymin (A-T or T-A, with RNA A-U or U-A) and Guanin-Cytosin (G-C or C-G). Three such base pairs (triplets) provide the code for an amino acid. All the many proteins of organisms are built up from around 20 different amino acids, whose sequencing determines the protein's specific quality. Proteins, like genes, are also subject to a universal ordering principle in this building block sequencing which is reminiscent of a text.

Viruses can to a certain degree be considered as the primal words of this biological writing.

Genes are the bearers of information and this becomes ever more complex as development advances. With the human being for instance there are 150,000 base pairs per gene. With around 20,000 genes the human genetic material is made up of around 3 billion base pairs. There may be a few hundred or a thousand base pairs in the genome of a virus.

That nature has been working with such a universal genetic language since life first appeared has often given rise to far-reaching fundamental discussions, even going so far as suggesting a bio-philosophical manifestation of the biblical statement '*In the beginning was the word...*', which in this context takes on particular relevance. DNA does not have any enzymatic or active metabolic functions but only a kind of 'writing' or code that, in a manner of speaking, records the cell's memory. In the living situation, however, this code or 'archive' of the past is continually being updated or newly 'released' so that the DNA reading can be interpreted afresh in every life situation and adapted to the context.

The earlier perception that we are determined by our genes no longer holds true since the genes themselves are subject to a higher regulative principle that is dependent to a large extent on ourselves and our behaviour. We are of course to some extent defined by our genes but the opposite is also true in that we are continually working on and transforming our genome through the way we think, feel and act. As the most recent research demonstrates people with anxiety disorder for example exhibit epigenetic changes which can be reversed after four weeks of cognitive behavioural therapy.[3]

We can therefore directly influence our genes.

Only a tiny proportion of all viruses is currently known. Gigantic genetic data banks now exist across the world, where the genetic codes of innumerable organisms are stored and yet science is continually being surprised by the appearance of vast numbers of unknown genes especially those of viruses. Some four billion viruses rain down from the atmosphere each day upon every square meter of the earth and of these more than 90% are completely unknown.[4] Soil bacteria as well as higher organisms absorb these viruses and so can change themselves genetically or develop further – in terms of immunology for instance. With every breath, we take in thousands of these viruses. A leaf of lettuce contains a billion viruses, a millilitre of lake or sea water can have up to 100 million viruses and even drinking water is bristling with these entities. The way in which viruses interact with our organism under healthy conditions remains largely unresearched, however, and the rapid advance in scientific knowledge will no doubt bring many surprises.

A recent analysis of the skin virome of 16 volunteers taken from 8 different parts of the skin, revealed several million different viral gene sequences which, like bacteria, show significant differences between the individuals as well as between the chosen skin areas. The colonisation of each person with countless different micro-organisms is highly individual. Amazingly, 94.8% of viral genes analysed were completely unknown[5] - that is they possessed none of the genetic properties that we are familiar with in other natural contexts.

Human skin is colonised by around 10 billion bacteria and about ten times as many viruses. This is also true of the mucosal lining of the intestinal tract, the air passages and the urogenital system. All these micro-organisms are in the first place not pathogenic; on the contrary they are intimately connected with our metabolic and regulatory processes and without them we could not survive. Research into the particular physiological importance of viruses is only just beginning.

One of the most important scientific discoveries of the last decades is that our entire genome was originally created from viruses.[6] This means that, as the primeval 'raw material' of the genetic code, viruses not only form the basis of our physical existence but are also the active biological agents for genetic innovation, variation and flexibility. Hence they play a key role in developing biodiversity and the variety of species on our planet – an understanding that is only slowly gaining traction because it shakes the foundations of the modern Neo-Darwinist concept of evolution.

The currently accepted teaching rests largely on the so-called Modern Evolutionary Synthesis theory according to which organisms evolve through chance genetic mutations. This leads either to advantageous new characteristics which are then retained or to detrimental qualities which are subsequently eliminated through natural selection – this is the theory up till now. The idea that genetic evolution involves biological communication on the basis of viruses is still a rare perspective.

The one-sided yet still widespread perception of viruses as parasitic and disease-causing toxic entities, is an over-simplistic understanding. The fact that in rare cases the absorption of viruses is associated with symptoms of illness is due to the fact that our physical, genetically-based organism, like all forms of life, is in a continuous process of development and that some developmental steps are difficult and cause crises. This is a universal law. In this sense the viral residues found in our genome can be seen as a form of sediment arising from the innovative processes of evolution.

We must also bear in mind that viruses, unlike other organisms, can very rapidly change themselves genetically – this is known as mutability. It means, however, that mutation does not only occur by chance at a specific 'place' in the genetic code but that viruses are altogether the 'world champions' of genetic mobility. They can take up, reject, replicate, mutate, transfer and recombine genes. It means they can also split genetic sequences and re-assemble them so that new characteristics emerge. We should not imagine that viruses are as genetically stable as say rabbits or flies. For example, the AIDS virus which, like corona and flu viruses, belongs to the group of RNA viruses, can change with '*breathtaking speed..., to the extent that after 2-3 years the original strain can no longer be distinguished from among the millions of differing and competing successors*'.[7] Of the approximately 10,000 nucleotides of an HI virus, ten mutate on a daily basis.[8] This also means that virus characteristics are continually changing.

The globally widespread fear of a supposedly new coronavirus is based on the concern that with Sars-Cov-2 we are dealing with a dangerous mutant version of this age-old virus which is unbelievably aggressive and could cause millions of deaths. Such an assumption may serve to feed the collective fear mongering but lies far away from reality. The effect that a virus may have depends in the first place on the organism and its immune system.

The Spanish flu with its 50 million deaths was the horror picture or highly effective tool used to stimulate collective fear when the horrific prognoses were being developed at the start of the current pandemic because its cause was assumed to have been an erratic and deadly virus mutation. A more precise analysis, however, shows that this flu epidemic, like many other mass infections, was due in large part to the widespread breakdown of the human immune system after years of war, fear and a massive burden of stress.[9] The subsequent genetic sequencing of the Spanish flu virus revealed a common influenza virus with several mutations such as are found each year, but there was nothing abnormal, however, that might indicate a 'killer virus'.

This high mutability is one reason why we are continually having to deal with new viruses. It is UV radiation in particular that causes the viral genomes to break down into numerous fragments which then spontaneously reconstitute themselves into new viruses with new properties.[10] This process is referred to as Multiplicity Reactivation[11] and is comparable to the basic processes of DNA and RNA repair which are continuously occurring in all living cells. It is the UV portion of 'living' sunlight in particular which contributes to the high mutability of viruses. In Indonesia people often fill polyurethane bottles with water that is often highly contaminated with microbes and leave them out in the sun for a few hours to produce drinking water of good quality. This procedure referred to as SODIS (solar disinfection) is also recommended by the WHO. This does not sterilise the water but the sunlight appears to have a health-inducing effect on the microbial constituents. It is an aspect which also throws light on the much discussed issue of mask wearing. Strenuous physical activity that results in sweating and a faster breathing rate as well as high ambient temperatures cause masks – especially those which are dark in colour – to provide veritable breeding grounds for unsavoury microbes and fungi. They are then taken in and then tumble out while breathing and speaking.[12] As is well known, growth that occurs in dark moist areas (mould, fungus, pests) is less appealing than when it grows in the sunshine and fresh air. It doesn't need a microbiologist to recognise this.

In this connection another important phenomenon should be mentioned regarding our understanding of viruses. We assume almost as a matter of course that the cause of a virus' behaviour *lies in the virus itself!* The virus is made out to be an active agent when in accordance with the old enemy cliche, we refer to the virus as attacking, infecting or mutating. This overlooks the fact that a virus is only what the organism makes of it. A virus without a host, that is without a living surrounding, has neither function nor significance. The virus can only be effective in relation to the life processes in which it is embedded. Whether a virus is taken in by an organism or not is up to the organism and not the virus. The way it behaves within the cell, whether and how it reproduces, when, how and where it activates which parts of its genetic material, whether it is destroyed, excreted or remains dormant in the cell – all this depends less on the virus itself than on the organism as a whole and the condition in which it finds itself. The perception of the virus as an enemy is due to the subject-object relationship of host and virus being confused. A virus is only as aggressive as the organism allows it to be.

We still know very little about the natural significance of viruses for the health of human beings and nature. This is because we are still so strongly enthralled by the image of the virus as an enemy. We simply have no direct perception of these entities and have to rely on indirect, abstract and often questionable means of verification. The 'facts' gleaned in this way are interpreted by a one-sided pathogenic approach and then swallowed whole. This allows the secret world of the virus to be misused in order to project into them objects of fear which are not there. Arbitrary explanations permeated by a psychology of fear grow from the soil of this half-understood knowledge and bring about the awful confusion we are experiencing today. It is hard to imagine a science containing more contradictions than that associated with covid-19.

Against this background we will now address the PCR test upon whose reliability and purpose the entire management of the Covid-19 pandemic with all its drastic measures has been based.

The PCR test

The principal scientific tool for diagnosing SARS Cov 2 has been the PCR test. Without it there would be no basis on which to declare a pandemic and therefore no scientific foundations for the drastic measures being imposed across the world. The entire epidemiology relies primarily on this test but very little is generally known about the way it works nor its lack of reliability. The questions that arise with regard to its validity will now be considered more closely.

The PCR test was developed in the 1980s by the American biochemist Kary Mullis (1944-2019). for which in 1993 he received the Nobel Prize. The test was originally developed as a genetic diagnostic tool, for instance for inherited diseases. It is what made the deciphering of the human genome – the Human Genome Project – possible. From the beginning Kary Mullis warned against using the test for the microbial diagnosis of infectious diseases[13] and with good reason, as we shall see.

The test involves taking a swab from the mouth and throat where the virus is suspected. On such a cotton swab you will of course find thousands of different viruses and bacteria because all the surface areas of our body are colonised by billions of them. A certain procedure is then used to extract the genetic material of all these viruses. We then have a solution containing a colourful mix of genetic material from which, with the help of so-called primers, the sought-for sequence is 'cut out' (more on this later).

This confronts us with the first problem, however, namely that of contamination. Today we know that on the mucous membranes of *healthy* people innumerable viruses are found, including pathogenic ones, and that in most bacteria viruses are also living. These are known as bacteriophages. The so-called aerosols, referred to as viral transmission agents, are present more or less everywhere and always colonised by various viruses as well – both outside in nature and indoors. Even the process of extracting and handling the swabs makes contamination unavoidable – this is a widespread problem in virology and a frequent source of error which has already led to many mistakes and misdiagnoses. In a US laboratory in 2006 for example, viruses from mice were found in cultured human prostate cancer cells that were then used for research throughout the world and not only 'infected' the laboratories but also falsified the PCR test. This meant that for six years more or less meaningless research was carried out to 'prove' that prostate cancer is caused by viruses, which then turned out to be a fatal mistake due to a simple case of contamination.[14]

Another key problem in the diagnosis of viruses is so-called purification, the isolation of a virus, which is the prerequisite for determining whether the virus is the assumed pathogenic agent. The coronavirus is around 150 nanometres in size (1 nm = 1 millionth of a millimetre) and can only be made visible using an electron microscope. A labour-intensive process is then followed to produce a precious metal or carbon image of the object without which nothing can be seen. Bacteria can be easily identified and single specimens observed using an optical microscope.

With viruses this is not possible. A virus cannot be extracted and investigated because it cannot be seen. And if it is made visible using an electron microscope further research cannot be undertaken because the image produced says nothing about its properties in the same way as a photograph taken of a glass of red wine reveals nothing of its quality. In order to prove conclusively that a virus is responsible for a lung infection, for example, it would be necessary to carry out a post-mortem examination of the deceased patient, extract some lung tissue and prove that the same virus is present in this tissue in significantly larger numbers than other viruses. This, however, has only very rarely been achieved. In places where such post-mortems are carried out in large numbers, such as at the University clinic in Hamburg-Eppendorf, chronic underlying conditions (lung disease, asthma, coronary heart disease, diabetes etc.) were found in every case. Seven out of 12 autopsies of those who had supposedly died of covid-19 had deep vein thrombosis, four died as a direct result of a lung embolism where a causal relationship to the virus is unknown. It was certainly possible to identify the RNA of Sars-Cov-2 in the lungs of those who had died but the presence of other viruses was not investigated.[15] A broad spectrum of potential pathogenic viruses would then certainly have been found, all of which could have been considered as the cause of death.

Focusing on one specific virus as the sole cause of a deadly illness is in principle highly problematic. The statement 'corona death' must therefore always have a question mark behind it, especially since most patients do not die of viral pneumonia but of a bacterial super infection which is in turn dependent on the general condition of the person and not on the virus alone. It is then often no longer possible to detect the virus in the case of such fatalities.

To obtain a genome sequence the virus would need to be completely isolated – which is not possible in any reliable way – and the sample taken would have to contain no other RNA structures (from the lungs or other micro-organisms). There can be no such certainty, however. We can isolate specific virus proteins or viral genetic sequences, but we cannot prove that what we have isolated is directly responsible for an illness.

The PCR test only finds what we already know.[16] We have first to know the virus and its genome – which as we have shown we cannot do for sure – in order to calibrate the test. In other words, the test does not measure an objective pathogen but something which I have defined as such without knowing whether it is true. A clearly defined base sequence is required for the PCR reaction to take place[17], which it is assumed originates solely from the specific virus in question and that this virus alone is responsible for the illness.

Because of the high level of genetic flexibility and mutability among viruses, we cannot exclude the possibility of the PCR test picking up viral fragments, inactive mutants, dead viruses or other RNA structures which, although containing the sequence being looked for, have no relevance in terms of an infection.

A patient who catches and dies from pneumonia in a hospital and who has previously tested positive for coronavirus, is recorded as having died of corona. Had he been tested for the influenza virus, which is not usually done, a positive test result would in many cases also have been found and the patient would have had to be recorded as dying from influenza.

One of the main pitfalls of the PCR test is that it is so sensitive that it reveals things that we do not know if they have any relevance to an illness. Christian Drosten, the virologist who is now well known in the media, was asked about the PCR test during an interview about the MERS epidemic (Middle East Respiratory Syndrome) of 2014 which broke out in the Arab world and was also caused by a coronavirus (MERS-Cov):

'... the method is so sensitive that it can identify a single genetic molecule. If such a pathogen for example were to be

found lying dormant in a nurse all day in the mucus membranes of her nose, she would be identified as a MERS case without being ill or even being aware of it. Where previously only critically ill patients were recorded in the statistics, those with very mild symptoms and even completely healthy people are now included. This is what explains the surge in cases in Saudi Arabia. This is further exacerbated by the sensational reporting of the local media.' (Christian Drosten)

Question: Do you think that the media has an influence on the figures announced

Drosten: *Throughout the region there is virtually no other subject discussed in the TV news bulletins and newspapers. And even the hospital doctors absorb this news. They then think they must shift their focus towards this illness which up to now has been very rare in Saudi Arabia. Medicine is also affected by fashion.*

Question: 142 deaths must be taken seriously though.

Drosten: *Of course. But the 142 deaths occurred over several years, they are not all from the current outbreak. I fear that the current increase is rather because there is a heightened awareness. It is no different in this country. If the 'Bild Zeitung' or the evening news reports on the outbreak of a particular virus, the number of lab tests will increase significantly. This is simply because doctors are then more aware and look out for the reported pathogen in a more focused way.*

Question: What do you think should be done?

Drosten: *It would be very helpful if the authorities in Saudi Arabia would return to the previously accepted definition of the illness. For what is of immediate interest are the genuine cases. Whether asymptomatic or mildly infected health care workers really do carry the virus, is for me questionable.*

Even more questionable is whether they can pass it on to others. The health minister's new advisory group needs to distinguish more strongly between essential medical diagnosis and scientific interest.

Question: Could not the WHO give more guidance?

Drosten: *The WHO is only able to make recommendations regarding the recording of cases but this is not legally binding. In the case of SARS for example they only recommended registering the cases with positive antibody tests.*

Question: And what does that mean?

Drosten: *Our organism is continually being assailed by viruses and bacteria. They often get no further than the skin or the mucus membrane barriers of the nose and throat. There they are successfully repelled before they can do any harm. Only when pathogens manage seriously to infect the body does the immune system develop antibodies. If antibodies are present, it means that the human being has in fact had an infection. Such an antibody test would make it much easier to distinguish between scientifically interesting and medically relevant cases.*[18]

What Christian Drosten expresses here could be described as common sense medical expertise because he begins with what is medically relevant and not from a questionable test which, though perhaps scientifically interesting, serves only to make the world crazy. Why he now takes a different view would need to be explained.

Whether a virus is the cause of an illness depends primarily on the virus burden, that is the quantity rather than the presence of a virus. Illness is only caused by a virus if it proliferates, and this is not something measured by the test.

There is a further problem with microbial diagnosis in that we cannot prove that a particular germ is *not* present. Complex analyses of the human virome have discovered that many so-called pathogens can be found in completely healthy people: Measles, Herpes, Zika, Noro and, yes, even AIDS viruses have been found in the human gut.[19] During the 1980s AIDS epidemic in South Africa more than 50% of the population in certain regions tested positive to HIV with the PCR test and the prognosis was for a million deaths. In reality, however, the death statistics over the following years showed no significant change; on the contrary, in parts of Uganda where according to WHO estimates wholesale decimation due to AIDS was threatened, the population most affected by the epidemic actually grew by 3.1% per year.[20] The coffin builders didn't experience any upturn in the market either.

The reliability of the tests is praised in terms of its sensitivity and specificity. The sensitivity of a test means the number of infections[21] the test accurately finds. If for example I have 100 infected people and the test reacts positively to 95, the sensitivity is 95%. The rate of false negatives is therefore 5% because the remaining 5 would not have been correctly read by the test.

The specificity describes how many *healthy*, non-infected people were correctly identified. If I test 100 healthy people and get 98 accurate negative results the specificity of my test is 98% and 2% would be false positives.

A quality assessment study of 463 German laboratories testing SARS Cov 2 produced a sensitivity of 97.7% to 98.8% and a specificity of 98.6% which at first sight suggests a relatively high degree of reliability.[22] These figures apply to tests carried out under optimum laboratory conditions in which the danger of contamination and sources of error are minimised. If, however, the tests are carried out in a GP practice or at airports it will look rather different. According to a report published in the British Medical Journal (BMJ) the sensitivity and specificity of tests done outside clinical laboratories falls to around 70% and 95% respectively.[23] With a cold caused by other viruses the specificity also drops to 92.4%. This means that 7.6% of those not infected with corona will nonetheless be included as such because the test confused other viruses with SARS Cov 2.

The basic principle is that: The lower the frequency of an infection in the whole population at a given time (prevalence), the higher the specificity of the test must be if it is to have any meaning. If out of 100,000 people, 1,000 are infected, it means that 99,000 are healthy. If the test only recognises 98.6% of those who are healthy it means that 1.4% of them, or 1386 people, are false positives. This means that more false results have been produced than correct ones. If only 100 out of the 100,000 are actually ill – which is closer to the reality regarding covid-19 – then the quota of false test results (1399, corresponding to 1.4% of 99,900, instead of 99,000 healthy test persons) is 14 times higher than those who are actually ill (100).[24] The figure of 1386 therefore relates to the calculated example with a prevalence of 1000 infections per 100,000 inhabitants while the figure of 1399 relates to the more realistic prevalence of only 100 per 100,000 inhabitants.

'We can assume there is currently a SARS Cov 2 prevalence of 0.025% as determined by the PCR test. This figure is arrived at from the daily count of new infections (around 1000), the population of Germany (around 80 million) and the factor 20, because the PCR test demonstrates the presence of an infection for an average of 20 days. Such a low prevalence of 0.025% means that even a test with 99.9% specificity will result in significantly more false positives than true positives. Only if the specificity reaches 99.99% can the tests yield reasonably useful results.' (Dr A. Sönnichsen) [25]

In other words, this mass testing is pointless and only causes utter chaos.

'In its most recent statement the Society for Evidence-Based Medicine demonstrates very clearly that the approach taken for combating the pandemic has in many areas distanced itself from basic scientific principles and hence from evidence-based medicine and that it has become highly politicised.' (Dr H. Matthes) [26]

Even the Deutsche Ärzteblatt, not known for being particularly critical, said of the positive predictions of the test:

'With 0.30 it is shockingly low – 70% of those testing positive are not positive at all but are nonetheless required to quarantine.' [27]

We must therefore remember that the whole story of the pandemic is based upon a highly questionable test.

The increasing numbers of tests undertaken in Germany (from March 2020 the number of tests steadily increased and between August 2020 and May 2021 more than one million were being carried out each week) had the logical consequence that the number of those testing positive – not ill people! – rose dramatically despite infection rates remaining steady or even falling. If more are tested, more will be found. If when presenting the daily figures no comparative ratio is ever given – those testing positive in relation to the total number of tests carried out – it is effectively deliberate deception. If I carry out 100,000 tests one week and discover 50 new infections and then in the following week carry out 200,000 further tests and find 80 new infections, it is not the number of new infections that have increased (they have in fact fallen from 0,05 to 0,04), but the tests. That it is the Bild-Zeitung[28] of all papers which has to explain this deception does not say much for the general approach to truth in our media. It is extraordinary how systematically this mistake regarding increasing infection rates is being promoted in the news bulletins. It is always important to remember, however, that these 'new infections' are rarely about illnesses caused but rather about test results.

The fact that the positive cases – that is the number of those testing positive in relation to the number of tests carried out – increases significantly during the autumn and winter months is a perfectly normal seasonal effect because this is when colds and flu generally increase and when more coronaviruses are to be found.

The principle behind the test is to duplicate the tiniest amounts of the previously defined viral DNA sequence until it is measurable. A fluorescent dye is used which accumulates on the DNA. By measuring the signals given by the dye with each duplication (amplification) the quantity of genetic material present (CT or Cycle Threshold value), can be calculated. The fewer the duplications needed to receive a signal, the heavier is the virus burden and therefore the risk of falling ill and infecting others, i.e. the infectiousness of the one being tested. The critical factor determining the viral load is the immune system or the level of stress a person is under.[29]

10-fold duplication gives me approximately a thousand times the amount, 20-fold duplication a million times and with more than 30-fold duplication the 'genetic fragment' is multiplied more than a billion times. Were I to receive a signal only after 40 duplications it would mean that the amount of the molecule being sought is only present at a 'homeopathic' level. There is now a discussion about how many PCR duplications should be carried out if the test is to make any sense at all. This question was recently addressed comprehensively in the New York Times:[30]

'Any test with a cycle threshold above 35 is too sensitive,'

said Juliet Morrison, virologist at the University of California, Riverside. *'I'm shocked that people would think that 40 could represent a positive .... a more sensible limit would be 30 to 35,'* she added. Dr Michael Mina, epidemiologist at the Harvard T.H. Chan School of Public Health, went further, saying he *'would set the figure at 30, or even less.'*

The threshold cycle is generally set at 40 today but this is often not stated explicitly when results are published; instead the test is simply presented as positive or negative.[31] This would be essential information, however, for determining the virus load and whether the person tested poses any risk of being infectious since at 40 there is virtually none. The C.D.C.'s own calculations suggest that it is extremely difficult to detect any live virus in a sample above a threshold of 33 cycles.[32]

'It's just kind of mind-blowing to me that people are not recording the CT values from all these tests — that they're just returning a positive or a negative,' said Angela Rasmussen, virologist at the Colombia University in New York (NY Times article, cited above).

According to Dr. Mina, of those who tested positive in Massachusetts, 85% to 90% would have been negative if, instead 40 cycles, the more realistic threshold value of 30 had been taken.

We can therefore see that there is a hidden leverage point which allows the pandemic to be arbitrarily manipulated in an upward direction.[33] It is a process which has occurred repeatedly as numerous other examples demonstrate. In 1992 the number of AIDS infections – or more accurately the number of positive HIV tests using PCR – had already reached their peak and were already declining when the definition of AIDS was changed. Until that moment a person was deemed to have AIDS if they had a positive PCR test and the number of T cells in their blood was below 100 per µl. It did not require any symptoms of illness. A reduction in the number of T cells can have many other causes which are not related to disease. That is why in Canada, for example, the number of T cells as a criterion for diagnosing AIDS was discontinued.[34] In 1993 the definition of AIDS was redefined by the CDC. Those were defined as having AIDS who had fewer than 200 T cells per µl of blood. This meant from one moment to the next the number of AIDS patients in the USA doubled, with all the serious consequences for those affected.

Something similar has been observed over many years with regard to high blood pressure, diabetes and high cholesterol levels; blood pressure thresholds and those of blood sugar and cholesterol were successively reduced, which led to the generation of millions of new patients and a corresponding increase in the sales of the relevant medicaments.[35]

With these tests and their interpretation we enter territory which is hard for ordinary citizens to fathom or understand. A complicated scientific process and level of exactitude is implied which does not in fact exist. So long as there are no characteristic symptoms for covid-19 we actually have no idea what we are measuring. With measles we can easily check the reliability of a test by looking to see whether the patient who has tested positive displays the typical symptoms. If more than 80% of those who test positive display no clinical symptoms or indicate that they are not ill at all, then the test doesn't work.

It has repeatedly been stated that a disturbed sense of smell and taste are typical characteristics of covid-19. However even this is deceptive since most pathogenic viruses are neurotropic, which means they can also affect the nervous system. The brain as the central organ of the nervous system can succumb to virtually all the usual viruses (herpes simplex, varicella zoster, Ebstein Barr, measles, mumps, rubella, enterovirus, ESME (Early Summer Meningoencephalitis) as well as influenza viruses which, to a greater or lesser degree, can always result in neurological symptoms as well as disturbances to the senses of smell and taste. If therefore I show symptoms of flu, my senses of smell and taste are disturbed and I have a positive SARS Cov 2 test result, it doesn't necessarily mean that I am sick with covid-19. It could just as well be some other influenza virus which nobody has yet tested for. What is new with covid-19 is in the first place the test, not the illness!

Never in the history of medicine has there been such an intensive and world-wide campaign against an illness as we are experiencing today. Millions of healthy people without any symptoms are undergoing mass orgies of testing for a supposed 'killer virus' using a test which is measuring something but we don't really know what it is. We are not able to grasp the significance of the genetic data that we obtain because we have no comparable data from the past. If we had made the same effort over the last ten years and investigated the viruses found in billions of nasal samples, what would we have found? We would certainly have found a plethora of corona viruses and countless mutations of them. In the year since the 'first' SARS Cov-2 virus from Wuhan was sequenced 4,000 mutations have been described. Up to now 13,000,000 new variants of the different SARS viruses have been entered in the central GISAID data bank[36] in Munich.[37] The first Wuhan virus also needs to be understood as one of countless virus variants. We would therefore expect to find innumerable different viruses in the samples taken from a million people, all of which might be considered the potential cause of an illness. Given this background of continuous change and diversity, it is hard to understand why one of these countless variants is currently dominating the world.

Countries like Thailand and Bhutan did not participate in this unfocused search for viruses but followed a path which has always proved itself in medicine. Tests were not carried out aimlessly on healthy people but only on those going to the doctor with symptoms. The patient was then assessed and appropriately treated. Only if the diagnosis was unclear would a PCR test be carried out (with a CT number below 35). Covid mortalities in Thailand and Bhutan were since the start of the pandemic, around one covid-19 death per million population, in Germany it was 866 during the same period.[38] With the overall death rate remaining unchanged it may safely be assumed that the majority of deaths from covid were the result of a new testing procedure re-defining the cause of death.

The immune system

A theme which has been criminally neglected throughout the corona discussions concerns the human immune system and the decisive role it plays in the handling of infections. Once again we find long outdated, one-sided thinking connected to a reductionist understanding of living processes manifesting itself. The isolated investigation of antibodies, T cells and other immunological factors without considering the socio-psychological, ecological and individual-biographical aspects ignores the single most important factor that determines a healthy immune system, namely ourselves. The immune system depends to a large extent on our own capacity for self-regulation, our social relationships and motivation in life or sense of meaningfulness.

A meaningful life is a healthy life, even if there are physical incapacities. This is the basic principle of salutogenesis as Viktor Frankl (1905-1997) has demonstrated in his biography. Chronic fear, social isolation and the experience of being devalued as a person all weaken our immune systems and are the most significant causes of illness that there are. Healing impulses can arise from the current crisis through an extended modern understanding of the immune system.

A key question which modern medicine needs to address is why there has been a steady increase in diseases relating to the immune system since the Second World War, particularly in the western world: In the case of cancer its reaction is too weak, with allergies it is too strong and with autoimmune diseases it attacks the body itself. In the USA nearly 50 million people suffer from some form or from several autoimmune diseases, of which there are some 80 different ones, and 60 million Americans are allergic or have asthma. The number of cancer cases in western industrialised countries has doubled since 1970.[39] There are half as many in the developing countries. During the same period of time the use of antibiotics, vaccines and fever-reducing drugs has increased at virtually the same rate. Whether there is a direct causal relationship is not precisely known but it is suspected at least, and the issue must therefore be looked at and discussed. The increasing numbers make it of high medical relevance.

An important issue connected to vaccines needs to be addressed now. Today we know that viruses are the oldest entities in nature, that all organisms existing in the world are colonised by countless viruses and that they have played a key role in the genetic regulation of all living organisms since the world began.

It is only in recent years, however, that studies have been undertaken to find out what viruses are actually doing in the context of *healthy* people. It has been astonishing to discover that on the skin and mucus membranes, in the lungs and in the intestines there are millions of different viruses including the so-called pathogenic ones. Over 70% were completely new, unknown viruses. Even in the blood of 8,000 healthy blood donors the genetic material of a total of 94 different types of virus could be found, with 19 of them being found in 42% of those tested. Amongst those found were: Viruses that cause smallpox, Hepatitis B and C, Herpes, papilloma viruses (HPV), which are linked to cervical cancer, AIDS viruses, yellow fever, early summer meningitis and other viruses.[40]

Viruses play an important role in the healthy human organism, which is perhaps not surprising considering the long evolutionary history shared by human beings and viruses. We know, too, that only once a certain number of viruses are present (the virus load) do they have any relevance in terms of illness – their presence in small numbers is quite normal. That is why so many people test positive to the PCR test without any illness symptoms. Viruses regulate the populations of micro-organisms in nature and enable the 50 billion or so bacteria which colonise a healthy human being to maintain a balanced ratio with one another. The so-called microbiome – all the micro-organisms living in a symbiotic relationship to human beings – is nowadays understood as an organ of the human being because of the numerous essential and important functions it fulfils in the organism. Viruses are part of this microbiome.

We can therefore no longer ignore the fact that by using antiviral vaccines we are interfering with the healthy processes of microbial and genetic regulation and in so doing increase the risk of autoimmune diseases. In the USA, where the policy of vaccination is very widespread, 15.9% of the population (41 million citizens) have antibodies that work against their body's own genetic material, so-called antinuclear antibodies.[41] There is a corresponding number of patients with one or more autoimmune diseases (type 1 diabetes, multiple sclerosis, rheumatism and others). The incidence of these conditions has been steadily increasing for years.

As elements of the microbiome, viruses and bacteria have organ functions and the 'battle' against these entities is not without consequences for our health. A responsible science needs to take account of these phenomena; otherwise the explanations will remain incomplete.

The link between antibiotic treatments and allergies has been demonstrated in many studies especially when carried out in early childhood.[42] A very recent Swedish publication shows that the risk of allergies and autoimmune diseases increases in a direct ratio to antibiotic use.[43] In cancer treatment the preventative and therapeutic effect of fever in the context of infectious disease has been documented time and again in numerous pieces of research for more than a hundred years.[44] Fever is not a symptom of illness but the expression of an immune response. It is justifiable to think that vaccinations have something to do with the apparent 'pandemic' irritation of our immune systems, and that by preventing fever symptoms a certain maturation of the immune system is prevented. Long-term comparisons between vaccinated and non-vaccinated children have not been carried out on any scale for ethical reasons lest there is a wave of infections caused by the unvaccinated group. The very few larger studies that do exist should cause us to take note and at the very least result in further critical questioning and more research. A recent questionnaire circulated by the Jackson State University in the USA amongst parents of vaccinated and unvaccinated children revealed the, in some cases, very serious consequences of vaccination in terms of allergies, neuro-dermatitis and autism.[45]

Millions of years of evolution have created immune systems of highly functional and immense complexity and it is generally agreed that the human immune system is the most differentiated and complex of all living organisms by far and that no one fully understands it. Pharmacological manipulation using newly formulated vaccines without sufficient knowledge of the individual immune constellation in particular is by its very nature beset with huge risks.

Quite apart from this, research carried out in the field of psychoneuroimmunology in recent years has discovered a great deal of evidence to show that human immune activity is negatively influenced to a considerable degree by socio-psychological factors such as stress, anxiety and feelings of worthlessness. This ought to give rise to a fundamental socio-political and socio-medical re-think.

Reducing everything to a simple enemy-friend or virus-antibody argument, as those promoting a global vaccination campaign do, is totally inadequate. We would therefore like to describe the complex nature of the human immune system and make it understandable.

First of all we need to understand that the immune system is continually learning throughout life and that we cannot separate our physical immunological from our psychological mental experiences, in the same way as no functional boundary can be drawn between the brain and the immune system – both are intimately and intricately interconnected.

The duality of body and soul, which goes back to the questionable postulate of the 17th century philosopher René Descartes (1596-1650), remains deeply embedded in scientific thinking, even though it no longer accords with our modern understanding. The still prevalent bio-mechanistic ideology which sees our bodily functions as mechanisms that can operate independently of the direction given by the soul-spiritual authority of the human I, has not reflected reality for a long time but nonetheless continues due to the growing commercial distortion of medical science and our health systems.

The key insight of psychoneuroimmunology is that our immune system makes no distinction between the kinds of stress it is faced with. Continuous confrontation with viruses, bacteria, toxins or cold causes the same level of stress to the immune system as the experience of chronic psychological stress through exclusion, humiliation or social indifference. Concepts such as powerlessness, overload and exhaustion apply to the somatic and the psychological fields in the same way. Those who still separate these two fields have not understood the nature of human medicine.

To gain a true understanding of how the immune system functions we must consider a basic principle of evolution which concerns the way organisms develop towards ever greater autonomy.[46] The ongoing direction of evolution in which human development is embedded also leads towards ever greater autonomy and freedom in terms of motoric, regulative and cognitive capacities and especially the capacity to emancipate ever more strongly from the given, pre-determined conditions of the environment. The current evolutionary process is about developing the human 'I'. The history of humanity like every individual biography is about grappling with the issue of freedom, independence and human rights. Evolution is not merely a matter of chance – it is no doubt that, too – but we can recognise a gesture in living organisms that leads towards ever greater autonomy and freedom.

Of all living organisms it is the human being who is most able to learn. This capacity for autonomous self-development means that the *evolutionary* principle is expressed in the human being. He can himself create the free human being which had not previously existed. A cat does not need to make a cat of itself, nature has already done that, but a human being only becomes what he should become through his own efforts. Our self-evolving I is the internalised principle of evolution, not a mere construct of the brain as it is often taught today but a unique phenomenon of nature, a soul-spiritual *reality*. Without this insight no human medicine will be possible in future.

With this background we now return to the immune system. An immune system that can learn, a so-called adaptive immune system, only began to evolve with the vertebrates. Previously the immune system was to a great extent genetically pre-determined, there was no possibility of adapting to new conditions. Insects have been flying against windowpanes for hundreds of years and do not understand that they cannot pass through them because they are unable to learn.

If we travel into a distant country and are stung by some exotic insect that our organism has never encountered before, our immune system will nonetheless find some way of dealing with the toxin because it is capable of learning just as the whole human being is capable of learning. Within our genome we have some 1000 genes responsible for the production of antibodies and they can produce millions of different antibodies. It is a learning process on a microbiological level that is no different from a mental learning process. A so-called genetic recombination process takes place in the immune cells, which means that the genes responsible for antibody production are transformed, they are effectively taken apart and reconstituted to create precisely the antibody needed for dealing with the insect poison. It then fits like a key into a lock. This is intelligence on an unconscious level – confront a problem, try to understand it and develop a solution or successful treatment. With immunological learning the same process occurs on a molecular-biological level as occurs with cognitive learning.

When you as a reader consciously follow this text, you will be taking in something new. In that moment you are creating thousands of new synapses in your brain in order that tomorrow you will be able to remember and recount what you have learnt to a friend. The synapses in your brain must therefore be able to create a pattern so specific that the exact content of what you have just absorbed can be reproduced. In order for the synapses to collate the subject matter in the right way, the genes of your brain cells must also be constituted anew. In other words, the same genetic recombination process is taking place as occurs in the immune cells so that you can process the new thoughts that you receive. This is one of the most astonishing processes of nature, namely that something which is entirely *new* and cannot be explained in terms of genetic determinism can be physically inscribed into our organism.

We therefore have a cognitive and an immunological learning activity and both are underpinned by the same biological-genetic processes. The genetic mobility and flexibility required for this is particularly pronounced in human beings because we have a far greater capacity for learning than any other creature. 98.7% of our organism is genetically identical to that of the chimpanzee but when it comes to the immune system and the capacity for learning there is a massive difference. The human being has far higher activity in terms of processing and transforming its genetic predisposition. The so-called editosome – the genetic element we use to update or bring out a new edition of the genetic text – is 35 times more active in the human being, especially in the brain, than it is in apes.[47]

The power at work in these things is our ego organisation; it is about being present, recognising reality, being aware of and working with what is happening around us, making it conscious and immediate, experiencing the contextual significance – being present and being active as an I. This power is continuously and actively present right into our micro-biology.

How we work with something new, how awake we are when we do it, is the same on the level of consciousness as on the immunological level, it is the power of the ego which expresses itself through the will to understand and engage with meaningful activity.

Health, according to the founder of salutogenesis, Aaron Antonovski, is not a state of being but a continuously evolving process. We are always surrounded with potentially sick-making influences that as ego beings we take up, process and through them develop new capacities. Just as our I has continuously to assert itself and sometimes even run against the stream, our immune system is also engaged in a continuous process of *learning*. That is why the intricate make up and functions of both our brain and our immune system are highly *individual*. The lasting nature and thoroughness with which we process external influences – they could be viruses but also propaganda and manipulation attempts – depends on how awake and aware we are i.e. with our *ego presence* of mind.

With this background we will now return to the corona crisis. We are confronted with something new. However, whether SARS Cov 2 really is such a new virus is open to question since according to a recent study carried out in Tübingen[48] most people who have not been infected have a background T cell immunity to SARS Cov 2. In this investigation blood samples were taken from 180 people who had been infected with the coronavirus and compared with 185 blood samples taken before the pandemic. While 100% of those who had recovered from the disease had active T cell antibodies, 81% of the blood samples taken before the pandemic showed an immunity against the supposedly new virus. It means in other words that previous contacts with other coronaviruses, which have been around a long time – they were first described in the 1960s – and have been found every year in numerous common colds and so-called 'summer fevers', were sufficient to develop at least a basic immunity. Although it did not give 100% protection it nonetheless reduced the risk of infection quite considerably and if any symptoms of infection appeared at all, they were generally very mild. Previous experiences of the bodily organism, like other experiences which we may have, enable us to deal more easily with problems and new situations.

Instead of the pointless and very expensive[49] mass testing programme it would have been wiser to test those in the vulnerable category for background immunity[50] on the basis of T cell counts and then, if necessary, take the appropriate precautions.

On the basis of these findings the fear of further waves is without any real foundation and there is no rational scientific argument for the planned mass vaccination campaign, for after all immunity in the population will gradually spread ever more widely and correspondingly reduce the danger of infection.

What can we do to strengthen the immune system

We have learnt that our immune system does not 'function' like some biological mechanism but is dependent to a high degree on ourselves and on individual factors. According to the concept of salutogenesis developed by Aaron Antonovsky, the three most important things for a healthy life are the capacity to grasp the context of life; its feasibility, which means being able to master the demands of life; and thirdly its meaningfulness, so that in leading our lives the realisation of certain ideal values can be experienced. At this point we can also add a fourth factor namely, authenticity.

There are people who lead seemingly 'perfect' yet unhappy lives. They fulfil all the tasks and goals that they set themselves in a committed way and very conscientiously and yet miss the of inner warmth experience of being in tune with themselves – something difficult to describe in a generalised way. The medical sociologist Ronald Grossarth-Maticek calls this the capacity for self-regulation, for living life well and with authenticity. He published a remarkable study about this. In the context of the so-called 'Heidelberg Intervention Study', a thousand people were observed for 20 years. At the beginning their physical data and state of health was recorded – weight, eating habits, inherited factors, smoking, sport, social interaction etc. In a specially developed questionnaire the participants were asked about their capacity for self-regulation. Twenty years later the assessment was carried out. As might be expected those volunteers with the greatest number of objective health factors as well as being good at self-regulation, turned out to be the most healthy while those who had neither had the poorest health. It is worth noting, however, that those who had no overall positive health factor, were overweight, did not engage in sport, had a poor diet and possessed inherited ailments etc. but who had a good capacity for self-regulation and were able to live their lives feeling authentic and well, had the same outcome after twenty years as those with all the positive factors who led an objectively healthy life but had a poor level of self-regulation.[51] A healthy life is therefore not only dependent on external factors.

Individual factors are normally hard to measure and therefore escape scientific statistical analysis, which can only operate using standardised, collective data.

A recently published study analysing the microbiomes of over 9,000 people aged between 18 and 101 relates indirectly to this. The men and women who were most healthy and had the longest life expectancy were those whose intestinal flora had during the course of time become most strongly individualised – that is they showed many characteristics that diverged from the norm. Interestingly this very individualised flora also offered the best protection against infections and other diseases. A lifestyle that is authentic is reflected in the microbiome and protects us from foreign infections in the broadest sense.[52]

Human life is individualised life. One of the most important insights for medicine in future will be the understanding that the human organism is so constructed by nature that it can only be healthy if 'occupied' by a unique individuality.

We come now to the general factors of health and how they influence the immune system. What simple measures are there for activating the immune functions?

It is known from numerous studies that all forms of physical activity, which always involve a heightened ego presence, lead to an increase in body temperature – walking in the mountains can easily raise temperatures above 38°C – and hence to an activation of the immune system. Even moderate physical activity can lead to a doubling of the total number of leucocytes in the blood and an activation of specific immune resistance. So, for example, the so-called phagocytes which as natural killer cells, eliminate viruses, bacteria and cancer cells, can increase fivefold in number. Regular activity maintains this effect over the long term and reduces the risk of infection, cancer, diabetes and much else besides.[53] Already spending time in the woods is sufficient to strengthen our immune system. As part of a study carried out in Japan people from the city were sent out into the forest where they simply relaxed, walked around and enjoyed nature. After one day the natural killer cells were found to have increased by 40%, after two days by 50% and the effect lasted for a whole month.[54] It is believed that terpenes, the natural etheric oils from trees that produce the typical forest smell, have an immune-stimulating effect. Regular walks in the forest are among the most effective measures for maintaining health.

Since the human being is in essence a social being good connections and lasting relationships play a central role not only with regard to psychological health. A meta-analysis of 148 studies into this subject indicated that the survival probability increases by 50% for all age groups when there is good and stable social contact between people.[55] Against this background the limitations on contact during the corona time can hardly be said to contribute to a state of general health.

We would not actually need any studies to recognise these connections. We are informed by our own feelings and general common sense. Alienation from nature is a main cause of illness today on all levels – psychological, physical and also spiritual. *Social distancing* to prevent infection may make sense with regard to mass gatherings or large events but for daily human interactions it is more likely to be counter-productive.

Risks of treatment

Many of the so-called corona-specific changes in the lungs for example should always be considered against the background of the particular concept chosen to treat covid-19. This fear-engendering illness is often treated with aggressive regimes of ventilation and courses of medicine (virostatic agents, cortisone, antibiotics) which in combination are not always beneficial to the patients. Premature intubation and ventilation, which is often recommended for covid-19 patients, often has fatal consequences for older people.[56]

A serious yet hardly acknowledged problem in the treatment of covid-19 concerns the drug Hydroxychloroquine. Although some laboratory (in vitro) studies show an antiviral effect, the most recent meta-analyses indicate that its use as a treatment for covid-19 is potentially harmful.[57] When used in combination with other active ingredients such as the commonly prescribed azithromycin it was frequently found significantly to increase the number of fatalities as compared to patients who were not treated with it.[58]

There is a very common and widespread genetic defect known as the glucose-6-phosphate dehydrogenase deficiency, also known as favism, which affects 7.5% of the world's population (over 400 million people). This genetic variant is so common because those who carry this gene are resistant to malaria and are therefore more protected and can survive better in regions where it is endemic.

In some parts of the world up to 20% of the population have this genetic trait (African Americans and Hispanics in USA, Latinos from South America, south-east Asians, inhabitants of the tropical regions of Africa and even Sardinia in Italy). Most of those affected are unaware of this genetic defect because they only become aware of it when, for example, they are confronted with the need to avoid beans and peas in their diet (favism comes from Fava, the Greek word for bean) and certain medicines such as aspirin. If, however, these people take anti-malarial medicines such as hydroxychloroquine, which in Italy and Brazil for example are used as a standard treatment for covid-19 and which Donald Trump recommends as the most important medicine for treating corona, some very serious side effects can occur such as haemolysis (the breakdown of red blood corpuscles) accompanied by fever and shivering fits. This causes micro embolisms in the lungs which can be confused with the clinical symptoms of a bad lung infection which in turn is then falsely diagnosed as covid-19 pneumonia.

Lung embolisms have been found remarkably often in corona patients on intensive care wards[59] and also in the post-mortem examination of covid-19 fatalities.[60] In these cases an investigation should have been carried out to ascertain whether the genetic defect was present or if chloroquine had been given. The medicament can also cause heart palpitations which in turn can also result in lung embolisms. Too little is known about these connections, even among doctors.

The higher death rates in the regions mentioned above need to be considered in relation to this therapeutic treatment which has been used by millions. The higher death rates in countries like the USA, Spain and Italy have multiple other causes (health care systems, social conditions, environmental causes, etc.) but a significant risk factor lies with this genetic defect in combination with hydroxychloroquine and other active agents for the standard treatment of covid-19. Normally a genetic test would have to be carried out before such treatment is undertaken in order to exclude the possibility of this genetic defect[61]; this, however, does not normally happen. This means that those affected did not die from corona as the statistics indicate, but from a treatment that had been mis-applied.

There are several international WHO reports (solidarity, recovery studies) in which 11,000 patients from 175 hospitals in Great Britain alone were in some cases given glaring overdoses of hydroxychloroquine with catastrophic consequences. The excess deaths occurring in countries like England, France, Italy and Spain reveal a shocking correlation with the use of these medicaments.[62] The studies mentioned were discontinued with the bland statement: '*These data convincingly rule out any meaningful mortality benefit of hydroxychloroquine in patients hospitalised with COVID-19'*. [63]

A euphemistic formulation which elegantly skirts around the fact that many people have died as a result of this treatment.

The manufacturing company Bayer gave 8 million doses of hydroxychloroquine to the German Federal Government, the USA supplied millions of doses to Brazil[64], where the genetic defect is very common. After initially promoting it strongly as a wonder drug the American broadcaster Fox News changed its tune in May and warned its viewers: 'This medicine will kill you.' [65]

Considering the serious consequences, these things *must* be openly discussed and investigated by an independent party because it concerns a great many human lives.

There were fatal consequences to the millions of false positive PCR tests carried out in the context of the AIDS epidemic. Not only were countless people driven to despair, confusion and suicide by supposedly being diagnosed with a deadly disease, the worldwide panic led to a confused over-prescribing of Azidothymidine (AZT) the tested medicament shown to be a 'lifeline'. AZT is virostatic and comparable to chemotherapy; it attacks genes in the cell. It has a retarding effect on the enzyme *reverse transcriptase*, which then led to the assumption that it would be suitable for treating retroviruses like HIV.

We have meanwhile discovered that reverse transcriptase is one of the oldest of enzymes and plays a key role in the genetic metabolism of all organisms. According to current understanding an active agent like this *must* have a direct effect on the basic processes of life. The initial positive effect is down to the fact that numerous viruses, bacteria and other parasites in which reverse transcriptase occurs, are killed off in the body giving rise to a seeming improvement. In the early days patients were given 400 mg every 4 hours, making it 2400 mg per day. We now know that after one or two years such dosage leads to severe bone marrow suppression and the destruction of immune cells because of its cytostatic effect. The patients then died with symptoms of an immune-deficiency syndrome which was falsely diagnosed, however, as being caused by AIDS.

A wave of fear now took hold in Europe as well, with many high profile figures apparently dying of AIDS while in reality they had succumbed to medical overdoses. This catastrophic error did not escape the investigations into AIDS and especially the so-called Concorde Study of 1994[66], whereupon the recommended dose was reduced from 2400 mg to 500 mg per day – to just a fifth! – and replaced using an alternative multi-therapy approach (highly active antiretroviral therapy, HAART) with the terse justification that the side effects were too strong. The fatal enormity of this disaster, too, was intentionally swept under the carpet.[67]

Almost prophetically Goethe has Faust saying to Wagner:

This was our medicine; the patients died,
'Who were restored?' none cared to ask.
With our infernal mixture thus, ere long,
These hills and peaceful vales among,
We raged more fiercely than the plague;
Myself the deadly poison did to thousands give;
They pined away, yet I must live,
To hear the reckless murderers blessed.
......
How blessed in whom the fond desire
From error's sea to rise, hope still renews!

Goethe, Faust Part I, Before the City Gate[68]

Alternative therapies for covid-19

It is often said that as long as we have no specific covid-19 remedy or vaccine there is very little that can be done in terms of prevention or treatment. '*Give cortisone, ventilate, keep the organs functioning, not much else can be done,*' said Prof. Hennersdorf from the Clinic of Gesundbrunnen in Heilbronn in an Interview with the Stuttgarter Zeitung on 21 November 2020. Since the start of the pandemic the very promising and much touted antiviral medicine Remdesvir has so far also shown no positive effects.[69]

That there are truly effective procedures in the field of integrated medicine is demonstrated by the positive results obtained in the specially dedicated corona ward at the Havelhöhe Hospital in Berlin. According to a statement by the Clinic's director Prof. Dr Harald Matthes in October 2020: [70]

'The initial large-scale studies into hydroxychloroquine and azithromycin, undertaken primarily in university clinics, were found even to increase death rates. The anthroposophical concept of therapeutic treatment which focuses on the strengthening of self-healing forces has therefore taken on greater significance. The important anthroposophic medicines used were iron in its meteoric form or as Ferrum metallicum praep., phosphorous, stibium as well as Cardiodoron® and Pneumodoron®, but also Bryonia (white briony) and Tartarus stibiatus (tannic acid). The results were very good

since up till now no covid-19 patient in Havelhöhe has died, given that otherwise there is a 30% death rate for covid-19 patients in intensive care.'

Apart from the treatments mentioned, the anthroposophic approach makes use of a wide variety of external applications including ointments, compresses, foot baths but also eurythmy therapy, dietary measures, soul-body harmony and much more.[71] Promising therapeutic concepts with homoeopathic remedies have also been reported from other countries.[72]

There are also a whole series of other highly effective remedies such as for example annual wormwood (Artemisia annua) whose anti-viral properties have been confirmed in a study by the Max Planck Institute. There is also Ivermectin which shows far more convincing results than that offered by vaccination. The effectiveness and above all the safety of this particular medicine has been demonstrated following many years of research and more than 4 billion applied treatments and yet 'officially' it is only recommended for treating covid-19 'in the context of research'. This simply shows that what really lies behind the pandemic policies is a long-term strategy of vaccination. Alternative ideas are not even considered despite very convincing evidence.

The use and risks of vaccinations

Never before have vaccines been developed for the whole world in such a short period of time. Under pressure from the global pandemic, the licensing procedures were drastically shortened. Yet, when dealing with vaccines intended for *millions of healthy people* it is particularly important that even more rigorous testing is carried out. With such high numbers of people being vaccinated it is likely that even the rarest side effects could ultimately have dramatic consequences.

'One serious adverse event per thousand of a vaccine given to 100 million people means harm to 100,000 otherwise healthy people...' (Prof. W. Haseltine, Harvard Medical School) [73]

With the currently favoured substances we are dealing with so-called gene-based vaccines whose long-term effectiveness for human beings has not been tested. Trials with apes have so far not yielded any relevant effects.

'We know all the candidates tested to date in non-human primates failed to protect any of the monkeys from infection of the nasal passages, the primary route of human infection.' (Prof. W. Haseltine) [74]

Vaccines made by the customary, classical procedures use deactivated viruses (dead vaccines) or weakened viruses (attenuated vaccines), viral proteins or even vaccination viruses impregnated with the SARS Cov 2 capsid protein. They stimulate an immune reaction by forming antibodies and T cells. The genetic vaccines by contrast contain the chosen virus gene in the form of mRNA or DNA which then serve as a kind of construction manual for the human cells. Genetic information is introduced which stimulates the production of virus proteins by the cells. This foreign protein then acts as an antigen in the organism, causing the intended immune reaction. It has, however, now been shown that the mRNA is primarily taken up on the inner surfaces of the cell vessels and by the blood corpuscles. This means that these cells produce the viral spike protein and are therefore attacked by the immune system with an increased danger of thrombosis.[75]

It is normal practice for every medicine to undergo a stringent regime of testing. Following initial laboratory and animal trials, a vaccine is subjected to a three-phase testing programme. In phase 1 it is trialled on a small number of volunteers to assess compatibility, side effects and distribution or metabolisation (pharmacokinetics) in the organism. A certain observation period is then allocated before a second dose is given. Then after further observation and follow-up – which, depending on available data, can extend over several years – the 2nd phase begins. The aim now is to determine the correct dose, how often and at what intervals the substance should be given to achieve the optimum result. This usually involves the testing of several hundred volunteers with special attention being focused on less common and delayed side effects. If it is shown that the benefits clearly outweigh the risks the 3rd phase begins, involving thousands of volunteers. The intention now is to see whether the vaccine is effective and prevents infection in the longer term, whether there are interactions with other medicines or if abnormal long-term immune reactions occur, such as for example a serious illness caused by other pathogens. Cross-immunisation in the body's own tissue can also occur leading to auto-immune reactions. This 3rd phase, which is most important for vaccine safety, normally runs for between four and six years. The entire period for developing a vaccine is therefore at least 8 years.

Bearing in mind this normal practice of carrying out meticulous, long-term vaccine trials the drastic reduction to less than a year must of necessity raise serious concern.

The long-term effects of vaccination cannot be known with any certainty because with highly individualised immune systems the effects of an irritation may only come later and the causal relationship to vaccination is not immediately obvious. Longer term effects of this kind, however, are entirely plausible because an irritated immune system can manifest itself in countless different response reactions and illness symptoms. The continually growing number of allergies and especially autoimmune diseases – currently numbering about 80 – should give rise to a fundamental rethink.

The first larger study into the tolerability of RNA vaccines was published in July 2020 in the highly respected medical journal The Lancet.[76] 543 trial participants received the RNA vaccine ChAdOx1 nCoV-19 and the following reactions to the vaccine were recorded: Tiredness and headaches 70% (340), muscle pains 60% (294), feeling unwell 61% (296), shivering fits 56% (272), feverish sensation 51% (250), fever over 38 degrees 18% (87), fever over 39 degrees 2% (8). Of the 54 people who received the covid-19 vaccine 45% (25) showed a temporary decline in neutrophilic granulocytes; these are important cells for non-specific immune resistance, a lack of which increases the danger of infection during this time.

As a control, a group of 534 participants was given Meningokokken (MenACWY), the already licensed vaccine against meningitis. In this case the various side-effects occurred far less frequently.

The age of those tested lay between 18 and 55. The risk of more serious harm from vaccine side effects increases with older people since they cannot so easily ride an adverse reaction. The protection offered by vaccines tends to decline in old age. So-called vaccine resistance starts around the age of 30 and steadily increases as the years go by. The available scientific data relating to older people is very sparse even though they are the ones most at risk from serious covid-19 complications and therefore in most need of protection. For pregnant women, children, people with underlying health conditions and other sensitive groups, these new vaccines have not been adequately tested.

A long-term risk relevant to these new vaccines concerns the development of so-called Antibody-Dependent Enhancement (ADE). Antibodies normally attach themselves to a virus, neutralise it and so prevent it entering the cell. The virus can then no longer reproduce, and the illness symptoms do not appear. Due to Antibody-Dependent Enhancement the opposite occurs; they attach themselves to the virus but enable it to enter the cell more easily, causing it to spread rapidly and develop serious disease symptoms. This is a recognised phenomenon occurring after vaccinations against measles, RSV (Respiratory Syncytial virus, a pathogen infecting the upper airways, often in children) and dengue fever. People who have been vaccinated against these illnesses and subsequently come in contact with the pathogen can develop ADEs leading to serious and sometimes fatal complications. Lasting lung damage was also observed in these cases. This problem can arise independently of the type of vaccine used. All vaccines targeted on the spike protein of the virus can cause abnormal immune reactions of this kind following subsequent contact with the coronavirus regardless of whether it contains the actual protein, mRNA, DNA or a viral vector. It is for this reason that no vaccines against MERS and SARS have been authorised.

'It seems a folly then to rush our way towards a vaccine in 2020 if it is likely to have only limited benefit to the population most in need and may put otherwise healthy people at risk. The risk goes far beyond the dangers a COVID vaccine alone may hold.' (Prof. W. Haseltine) [77]

What is most concerning here is that those being tested in the context of this study have not been made sufficiently aware of the risk posed by such delayed vaccine effects.[78]

And what about the protection offered by the vaccine, how long will it last?

There is generally no expectation on the part of vaccine manufacturers that the vaccines will provide life-long immunity.

The long-term immunological effect of vaccines is usually determined by the antibodies circulating in the blood, but this does not reflect the true state of immunity. There are essentially three levels to our immune defences. Many pathogens are eliminated when first coming into contact with the body. On the mucus membranes, in saliva and in lacrymal fluid (tears) the so-called lysozymes are formed and along with them immunoglobulin (IgA). These are generally sufficient for healthy people to resist pathogens. In these cases there is no significant increase in the number of antibodies and so those affected are often wrongly assessed as having no resistance. The antibodies which neutralise viruses only appear on the second level as IgG and IgM antibodies.

A third longer term immune capacity is developed by a certain group of T-lymphocytes, to which memory cells belong. As we shall come to see in what follows, an analogy to our inner memory function can be helpful in understanding the long-term immunological memory because even on a purely biological level they have much in common (see below). It is very important to form this conceptual linkage during this period where corona fear is rife in order to overcome the outdated idea that our immune system is merely a biological mechanism that functions independently of us. We do have a great influence on our immune system.

In the psychological realm we speak of active and passive memory. 'What have you done this year in the summer holidays?' That is something which everyone can usually describe immediately because it is still consciously present. This is to some extent comparable to antibodies which are present, active and can be immediately called upon. A question, however, such as 'What did you do on 5th July 3 years ago?' is unlikely to be so readily present. The person may not actively remember it but needs a nudge first, such as a photo from a trip to 'bring it all back'. This scenario corresponds to the memory cells which only wake up and become active in response to a particular stimulus such as renewed contact with a virus.

Against this background it is not possible to make generalised statements about vaccines, how long the protection will last or the immunological 'competence' of a patient without first knowing an individual's medical history and general state of health. Sensible decisions concerning vaccines are always made on an individual basis.

How does the immunological memory relate to an illness as compared to a vaccine?

In the memory experience of the body-soul complex an illness is usually retained better than a vaccine. By going through an illness, the human being *deepens* its connection with the organism (lying in bed, fever, aching limbs, feeling weak). This experience is not played out on a conscious level, but the body is nonetheless confronted with something new and, in processing it, gains a higher level of immunity and at the same time greater autonomy. The bodily substance is *individualised and penetrated* in much the same way as a person's development and life is affected by an important experience. A mother who was ill with measles, mumps or German measles as a child gains more experience on an immunological level than a mother who had merely been vaccinated as a child. This experience is passed on by the mother to the child who thereby gains passive immunity in the form of IgG antibodies. This so-called maternal passive immunity is significantly less long-lasting in mothers who have been vaccinated or, to put it another way, their immunological training has been less thorough.

The immunity produced by antibodies is known as sterile immunity because viruses are rapidly and completely eliminated by them or perhaps we should say, *processed* better. The immunity facilitated by T cells corresponding to passive long-term memory may also be called clinical immunity. It does not lead to the complete elimination of a pathogen but usually ensures that the course of the infection is very mild, if indeed there are any symptoms.

How meaningful is it to vaccinate against covid-19 and other infections of the air passages?

During the swine flu outbreak of 2009, 34 million doses of vaccine were made available in Germany. Of these around 4 million were used while the rest – almost 90% with a total value of 250 million Euros – had to be destroyed. Despite the very low vaccine uptake (only 5% of the population were vaccinated) the flu mortality figures of that year were among the lowest for 20 years. To put it bluntly: Apart from the enormous waste of money and a few hundred cases of vaccine-related narcolepsy, the vaccination campaign had no effect. In order not to repeat such a debacle with covid-19 the pressure to vaccinate was increased massively by threatening to take away long-term civil liberties and other repressive measures. With the help of sociologists[79] and psychological strategies (see below) ('vaccination is freedom', financial incentives and other tempting offers), vaccine uptake could be increased to currently over 60%. According to surveys (see previous footnote reference) 16% of the population categorically refuse the vaccine and 17% are undecided.

To vaccinate children with these totally untested substances without knowing the long-term consequences is to my mind a criminal act of reckless negligence.

According to meta-analyses carried out by several German universities[80] the risk of a child (0-14) dying from covid-19 was about 1:3.5 million. In other words, of the 14 million children living in Germany today 4 have died of a covid-19 infection and it must be remembered that even in such tragic cases there were underlying health conditions.

How great then is the statistical chance of dying from a vaccine-related complication?

The number of adult deaths associated with the covid-19 vaccine lies between 1:14,000 (ca 6000 recorded deaths per 88 million vaccinated people in Europe, as of 5th April 2021[81]) and 1:58,000[82]. It is of course impossible to prove a hundred percent causal relationship between vaccinations and deaths, just as it is to pinpoint the coronavirus as the sole cause of death in the case of a lung infection. The recorded statistics do, however, suggest that a connection to the vaccine is highly plausible. The longer term mortality rates resulting from the vaccination could well be far higher. This is because the irritation caused to our highly individual immune systems can have a great many unknown consequences and with the mRNA vaccines it has simply never been investigated.

The covid-19 vaccine causes acute reactions particularly among younger people in the form of fever, headaches, aching limbs and sometimes also shivering attacks. Taking the most favourable of the vaccine mortality rates for adults of 1:58,000, the risk of children dying from the vaccine is almost 60 times higher than from a corona infection. The way countless politicians dismiss such data when making their pronouncements can only really be explained by the massive lobbying campaigns undertaken by the pharmaceutical industry.

Another word about the so-called mutations.

It is fundamental that viruses affecting the air passages always mutate (see above). An important question here is whether vaccines make these so-called variants of concern appear more strongly. It is something that has already been suspected by a number of respected scientists such as the Nobel Prize holder Luc Montaigner[83] and the Irish immunologist Dolores Cahill. With antibiotics we already know about this 'home made' problem in that some 15,000 people die per year in Germany from multi-resistant bacteria. A lot of things in life only become enemies when we declare them to be so. Bacteria like viruses are important co-habitants of our organism and we cannot make them into enemies without risking collateral damage.

Israeli studies show[84] that at least two weeks after adults have received two shots of covid vaccine they have an 8 times greater risk of being infected by 'aggressive' mutations of this kind – in other words it is a similar phenomenon to that of antibiotic treatments. This finding was confirmed in a paper published by Public Health England in July 2021[85] about the covid delta variant that was so prevalent in England. It found that of 123,620 infected by the delta variant, 257 died (0.2%). Of these 92 (36%) were unvaccinated, 163 (63%) had received one or two injections and 116 (45%) were fully vaccinated. It clearly shows that significantly more vaccinated people died than unvaccinated – the precise opposite of what one would expect from a vaccine.[86]

The medium- and long-term risks associated with such entirely new vaccines have been inadequately researched especially with regard to children. We therefore have no idea what we are doing, and this is the height of irresponsibility. There are no rational reasons for recommending the vaccination of children; on the contrary there are likely to be more deaths than from covid itself. Making social interaction and going to school dependent on a child's vaccine status departs from any form of medical common sense – as the Bundesverband der Kinder und Jugendärzte (German federation of paediatricians) also emphasised in a public statement – but is an attack on the human dignity of the child which will undoubtedly increase the already serious psychological consequences. Who is going to take responsibility for this?

Contrary to a flood of alarmist forecasts, we had no excess mortality in Germany[87] in the corona year 2020 when without vaccinations, which one would actually have expected with the definition of 'pandemic'.[88] Since the fall of 2021, an increasing excess mortality has been emerging as the vaccination rate increased; it was 10% in September, 9% in October, 20% in November, and 22% in December 2021.[89] At the same time corona mortality declined, so the significant increase in excess mortality cannot be explained by the pandemic.[90] The mortality rates follow the frequency of booster vaccinations in a striking correlation.[91] (See figure below)

In a pandemic one would actually have expected the opposite: that there would be excess mortality in 2020 when without vaccinations and the opposite in 2021 after the introduction of vaccinations. Without a critical reappraisal of such alarming figures and without a public discussion about it, the introduction of compulsory vaccination is more than irresponsible, indeed it is basically a criminal measure because it ignores not only the constitutionally enshrined right to self-determination and physical integrity, but it also ignores a multitude of scientific facts and thus exposes the population to incalculable health risks.

Comparison between the course of booster vaccinations and excess death counts by week in four separate countries: Austria, Germany, Switzerland and Israel

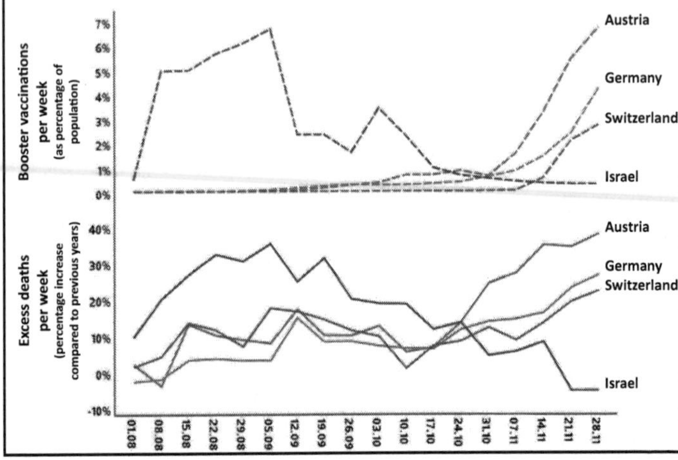

Fear and Power

The virus then, is not new. What is new is the global state of anxiety and an unprecedented interventionist approach which brings ruin to large sections of the global economy, greatly increases the problem of starvation in the third world, causes mass unemployment, cripples the cultural life, destroys millions of livelihoods, threatens basic freedom and human rights, uses all means to silence truth seeking journalism and ramps up fear across the world to pathological levels. And this is the main criticism from the point of view of immunology: Contrary to what is said, these measures do precisely nothing for human health. In the long run the damage caused will be far greater than the virus problem. 'Far more people will die as a result of the lock downs than from the virus,' said Gerd Müller (CSU), the German Minister for Development in an interview.[92] David Beasley, executive director of the UN World Food Programme spoke of starvation of biblical proportions as a result of the global measures against the coronavirus.[93]

With the best will in the world a sober diagnosis does not reveal an unusual level of infection or an increased death rate due to coronavirus in our society[94], uncertainty and anxiety disorders, however, are noticeably increasing.

Thanks to the opaque way in which epidemiological data was collected, it is hard at this point in time to see precisely whether regionally higher death rates are due to the virus or the lockdown measures.

Since the early 1970s when the policy began of opening up the health services to the free market and subjecting them to economic laws[95], fear has become the competitive motor driving what is now the largest economic sector in the world[96], and it is not difficult to see how it is being applied ever more successfully. Whoever wants to exercise power or make a profit needs to first stoke fear and then step forward as the 'saviour' who will rid people of that fear – with a vaccine for example. The corona crisis exists almost exclusively through fear. We will look at the psychological aspects more closely later.

Fear mongering has always been the most effective means for exercising power.[97] History is littered with examples of how ramping up images of the hateful enemy and presenting threatening scenarios has radicalised people, caused them to attack one another and engage in violence and terrorism. In the recent past there was the cold war which with the collapse of the Soviet Union, was replaced by the war on terror and the countless innocent lives that were sacrificed and now in a new era by the threat of a viral pandemic.

Interestingly we find that the institutions who are now managing the global pandemic are the same ones who previously were active in the campaign against terrorism and the threat of biological weapons. The Center of Health Security at the Johns Hopkins University, which has taken on such a leading role in the corona crisis and which has from the very beginning been releasing 'alarming' statistics concerning so-called new infections, was previously called the Center for Civilian Biodefence Studies. It was essentially a military institution which in the 20 years since 9/11 has kept the images of fear alive about the terrorist threat from bioweapons, smallpox and other killer viruses. During regular international conferences attended by high-ranking representatives from government, economic interests, pharmaceutical companies and the military, this organisation ran exercises to manage terror scenarios with millions of deaths in minute detail. The most recent crisis simulation took place on 18th October 2019 in a New York luxury hotel called Event 201. This time it was not a terrorist attack but the threat posed by a deadly coronavirus mutant that was simulated. A crisis management programme was designed, the individual measures of which bore a remarkable resemblance to those introduced in real life three months later.

> *'The significant thing about this exercise as well as the subsequent real-life situation was a conflation of fear, mass deaths, national emergency, over-extension of the state, restrictions on freedom, vaccines, pharmaceutical regulation and media strategy. More directly stated, a health emergency leads to a global demand for vaccines which in turn requires that corporations play a more active international policy making role in order to finance, produce and distribute them and that the inevitable resistance from the population is met with PR strategies and the media. That is what the exercise was about – and that is what is happening today.'* (P. Schreyer) [98]

It is clear to any observant person that the numbers are being manipulated and everything is being done here to maintain fear and panic at the highest possible level.

What does fear do to human beings and their immune systems?

In stress research we distinguish between so-called positive *eustress* and negative *distress*. *Eustress* means the increased stress resulting from a 'welcome challenge'. We become motivated, engaged, conscious, awake and can grow beyond ourselves. Or put another way, our ego is present in the way previously described. This kind of stress is healthy because we become active and even feel a sense of fulfilment, meaning and self-confidence. The immune system is then likewise positively stimulated, as when engaged with sport which although a lot of effort is required there is no fear or stress.[99]

With *distress*, it is the other way round: our ego withdraws under the influence of fear, powerlessness and helplessness. We are demotivated, feel out of control and confused. We have an urge to escape or else grow rigid. Such conditions, if they become permanent or occur regularly, can be poison to our immune system and hence to our health. A high level of the cortisol stress hormone can in the long term cause a so-called TH1/TH2 shift. An imbalance occurs between the various immune factors. The so-called TH1 system is repressed, certain messengers like the tumour *necrosis factor alpha* no longer develop sufficiently and the activity of the phagocytes declines with the result that there is greater susceptibility to infections and serious illnesses. By way of compensation the so-called TH2 system is strengthened, and this in turn leads to excessive antibody production and an increasing risk of allergies and autoimmune reactions.[100]

The increasing numbers of immune diseases, including the growing psychological problems in industrialised countries, has clearly got something to do with the increased level of collective stress caused by a society driven by a desire for growth and profits. Following the economic imperatives of increased efficiency, rationalisation and speed we have not only brought outer nature to the point of breakdown but also strained the internal ecology of the soul and immune system to the extent that an inner reflection on the true values of human culture is urgently needed.

The Real Crises

Climate change is advancing with worrying speed, alarming numbers of species are facing global extinction with unknown consequences[101], the world's oceans are increasingly contaminated with plastic waste, the reckless deforestation of rain forests continues despite the danger posed to planet earth, disease threats are increasing across the world due to ecological destruction and the gap between rich and poor grows ever wider creating a huge potential for social conflict.[102]

Since the beginning of the corona crisis the number of billionaires has increased worldwide from 2000 to 2700 and since March 2020 their assets have increased by 60% (!) to a level of 13 billion dollars (in May 2021). The world economy has simultaneously shrunk by 3.3% and 100 million people were pushed into absolute poverty as a result of the lockdown measures and forced to live on less than $1.80 (US) dollars a day. The consequence is that over the coming years death rates are likely to see a massive rise.[103] It is not only the pharmaceutical, digital and online businesses that benefit, the financial institutions are also reaping huge profits from the new wave of indebtedness arising from the corona investment programmes.

Compared to corona we have a huge number of preventable deaths across the world: 690 million people are starving and over 10 million die each year from malnutrition. Each day 15,000 children die of starvation, which could be prevented relatively inexpensively.[104] Instead it is being made massively worse by the corona measures[105]. With just one percent of global arms expenditure, currently running at nearly 2 trillion dollars, the problem of starvation could be solved. The eight largest food retailers paid out ten times more to shareholders than the UN would require to end hunger.[106] Worldwide 7 million people die each year as a result of air pollution, according to the WHO, in Germany alone 80,000.[107] Over 4 million die from diabetes which could be largely prevented with a healthy diet. 3 million die because of alcohol[108], 8 million from smoking, and 600,000 from drugs – about as many as died from corona in the first 6 months of 2020.

If it were really about protecting life and health, there would be far more sensible things to be done. But instead, the repeated lock down measures are increasing the hardship that millions of people are facing.

covid-19 as a global phenomenon is only one of many symptoms of a crisis in human consciousness. We are standing on a threshold which demands a fundamental re-orientation of our relationship towards nature, otherwise even worse catastrophes will follow.[109] The healthy way out of this crisis is not via a new vaccine but a new way of thinking.

Aspects of media psychology in relation to the corona crisis

Whoever has spent 30 years working as a doctor in a hospital will have experienced grave illnesses, suffering and death on a daily basis as well as serious infectious diseases, overflowing intensive care wards and – thanks to the reductions in staff imposed as part of the commodification of medicine – more and more highly stressed and exhausted co-workers.

Each year hundreds of thousands of patients die in German hospitals. They are mostly old people who at the end of their lives contract a lung infection and frequently have to go on a ventilator. Of the 900,000 deaths recorded on average each year in Germany only 23% die at home. This was also the case before the pandemic. The 50,000 deaths from pneumonia each year have often been redefined during the corona period using a new form of diagnosis.

The deaths that occur on a daily basis normally take place without any public awareness. This changed with the pandemic. For one and a half years images of intensive care wards filled to capacity, people dying and on ventilators as well as over-worked doctors and nurses, have filled the news bulletins each day, and these images have been presented within a completely new frame of reference, namely of the corona pandemic. A closer analysis of the absolute number of cases and deaths shows that nothing significant has changed, the images, however, were psychologically evaluated in a completely different way. They gained a new significance within the pandemic narrative. Colloquially this is known today as 'framing'. Countless soul patterns lying hidden in our sub-conscious are set off and begin to resonate through an experience or a word that we hear. A 're-processing plant' sounds quite different to a 'nuclear waste dump' and awakens quite other associations even though they refer to the same thing. Reprocessing suggests a solution, a waste dump the opposite. We evaluate death in the context of a plague very differently to a person of 85 who dies naturally of old age. If we are presented with numerous images of patients on ventilators under the headline 'mass deaths caused by the pandemic' patterns of fear and worry arise in us because the concept of a pandemic contains within it the concern that it could also affect me. Death is then no longer something individual but a collective happening.

The techniques of framing are being used in political propaganda in an ever more focused way and play a key role in the management of public opinion.[110] Becoming aware of and recognising the psychological patterning opens the way towards individual judgement and inner freedom. A basic rule of advertising psychology is that the most lasting effect comes about through continuous repetition. That is something known to power strategists throughout the ages. By continually repeating the same simple slogans (the betrayal narrative, hatred of Jews and communists, hero worship, leadership cult), the National Socialists succeeded in transforming a nation of 'poets and thinkers' into a murderous fascist state with countless accomplices and followers in a very short time. In the nineteen twenties the American tobacco industry, using a psychologically very sophisticated advertising strategy, was able to persuade millions of women to take up smoking and hence cause thousands to get cancer.

The phenomenon is known in psychology as the 'illusory

truth effect' – the more frequently a statement is heard, the more credibility it accrues even if to begin with the truth of the statement is less than convincing. The effect of this suggestive power of course depends on our consciousness and presence of mind, and it is often more comfortable to repeat an 'accepted' explanation than to reflect and make the effort to come to one's own conclusions. Frequently repeated statements and ways of thinking are much more deeply anchored in the brain. In neurobiology this is known as Hebbian Learning. The synaptic connections which form anew with each learning process, stabilise and consolidate themselves ever more strongly with each repetition. Unfortunately this also occurs with false assumptions and untruths. We all know how deep our ingrained habits lie and how difficult it is to change them.

As second basic principle of psychology is that advertising success does not depend on whether the object being promoted is genuine. If an advertisement for margarine shows a laughing happy family sitting at breakfast in a beautiful garden, the margarine has absolutely nothing to do with the happiness of that family. The continuous repetition of this blown up yet false association between family happiness and the margarine will nonetheless work unconsciously into our purchasing behaviour if we are not sufficiently awake to these things. In an industrial society where 'having' and 'consuming' occupy the highest position in terms of value, we have become so used to the 'imbecility' of these advertising slogans that we accept them as 'normal'. In doing so, however, we are corrupting our healthy sense for truth. Through this we are for instance conditioning our children to adopt self-harming behaviour which society will ultimately have to pay a high price for – we only need to think of the connection between the advertising of unhealthy food to children and the problems of obesity, diabetes and other metabolic conditions.

According to a recent study by Foodwatch[111] a child in Germany watches on average 15 advertisements promoting unhealthy food each day. 85.5% of these products are damaging to health. 15.4% of 3 -17 year olds are overweight (the last forty years has seen an eightfold increase). According to this study the estimated health costs are 400 billion Euros. In Germany alone there are 175,000 deaths associated with diabetes each year,[112] (the official figure for covid 19 deaths in 2020 by comparison was 30,000) which in the vast majority of cases could be reduced if appropriate measures were taken.[113]

Where is the public outrage and political concern for this? A ban on the marketing of junk food to children – just one of many examples – would be far more effective in the long-term than all the rituals of mask wearing and social distancing for which there is no scientific evidence and whose symbolic effect is to reinforce the ever-present sense of impending threat.

Economic interests clearly carry far more weight than maintaining human health. At a time of increasing digital connectivity through which the influence and extent of the psychological manipulation techniques grow ever greater, there is an urgent need for society-wide enlightenment. This concerns not only ethical values, our freedom and human dignity but also our health.

Why is the power of propaganda so great?[114]

Some common forms of psychologically conditioned human behaviour have developed over thousands of years during the course of evolution. This is because they make sense and have proved themselves time and again. We can take a simple example. When danger threatens in the form of a natural catastrophe or an enemy attack, people become fearful and look to each other for support because on the one hand it is easier to cope with the fear together and on the other because being together in an emergency offers a better chance of finding a solution. This is the reason why people who are sceptical of the corona narrative and ask critical questions suddenly become objects of hate for wide sections of society. No one listens to their arguments, instead they are judged as dangerous outsiders and a threat to the community because in the face of danger the all important 'solidarity in survival' is betrayed. It is, however, a false solidarity because it is driven not by human concern, insight and conviction, but by mere unconscious fear.

The more anxious a person the more likely it is that he will fall for the propaganda of fear. Clinical conditions of anxiety have increased massively over the last decades. The many hidden forms of anxiety that we all carry within us often only require a certain stimulus to be activated (this is known in psychology as a 'nudge'). Images such as the coffin-laden lorries in Bergamo that were instantly seen all over the world are particularly effective as media tools in terms of their shock effect. The power of such images – they were re-posted globally before anyone knew what they were really about – tends to overwhelm the common-sense perception of reality.[115]

Another very powerful example of unscrupulous propaganda was the 'incubator massacre' that was circulated globally by the media. The evening news showed a 'weeping nurse' who reported that in a Kuwaiti hospital Iraqi soldiers had come, ripped out babies from the incubators and threw them on the floor. That was also a highly effective psychological ploy that produced worldwide revulsion and hence international acceptance of the American invasion of Iraq. Only later did it transpire that the supposed nurse was actually the daughter of the Kuwaiti ambassador in the United States who had never worked in that hospital. The whole story was invented by

Hill & Knowlton, the US PR agency.[116]

Iraq's supposed weapons of mass destruction, referred to in 2003 by the American Secretary of State Colin Powell during a speech to the UN Security Council, also turned out to be fake – something that Powell later regretted, yet he remains co-responsible for the deaths of millions of people.

For two years we have been subjected to an endless barrage of fear messaging by the media regarding the threat posed by corona viruses. The enormous and continuous promotion of this propaganda by the media bears no relationship to the actual threat from corona viruses. It has, however, penetrated so deeply into the human sub-conscious that any criticism or counter arguments have virtually no chance, and even publicly available facts and truths are drowned out by the ongoing clamour of alarmism.

From a psychological perspective the suggestive power of this propaganda arises primarily through the reactivation of old patterns of fear – and we have been thoroughly and massively impregnated with this through our parallel media world. By the time they enter primary school children in the USA will have seen 8,000 murders and around 100,000 acts of violence on television. According to a research study, 25,000 murders and 439 violent acts against children have been shown on German television.[117] With every such experience the various fear patterns impress themselves more deeply, while causing on the other hand a certain blunting in terms of the toleration of violence. A current study being carried out by the German Federal Institute for Population Research (BiB) shows that the number of young people (16 to 19) with clinical symptoms of depression (requiring treatment) rose during the spring of 2020 from 10.4% to 25.2%.[118] It is not uncommon for depression to signal the onset of chronic illness. According to a study carried out by the University of

Hamburg Eppendorf the problems associated with the social integration of young people have also increased significantly. While before the pandemic 11% were affected, it is now 27%.[119] These are deeply worrying figures. Repressive social measures and the increased use of social media appears to have potentised their negative effects.

The search for lurid sensationalism upon which our commercial media thrives has produced in many fields a long-lasting and distorted perspective on reality with false enemy stereotypes, irrational fears, prejudices and much more. For example: On 26th February 2016, two months after the New Year's Eve event in Cologne, screaming headlines in the German media declared that two young Afghan refugees aged 19 and 26 had supposedly molested three young women outside a pizza shop in Kiel causing them to take flight followed by an ever growing number of refugees seeking to film them with their mobile phones. This news resulted in a massive hate campaign on social media with calls amongst other things to 'send them all packing'. Politicians, including the German president, sought to outbid each other on the evening news with expressions of outrage, which in turn incited millions of people to turn against the refugees.

What had actually occurred, however, is described by the 'Die Zeit' journalist Bastian Berbner in his book that is well worth reading, 'Stories Opposing Hatred'. Two 17 year old Afghans had blown kisses to three girls (aged 15, 16 and 17) with a few cheeky comments. That was all. There was no molesting, no filming and no pursuit. A scene which occurs on a daily basis in hundreds of school playgrounds was blown up into a sensational media event and into a nightmare for those affected. The cold war, terrorism, Islamism and most recently the pandemic threat are to a great extent also media-incited fear scenarios which have very little to do with the observations and daily experiences of ordinary citizens.

Many more awake observers of the corona narrative have seen no real evidence of what might be expected from a lethal pandemic. All the dire prognoses regarding mortality and the breakdown of supply chains have never materialised. From a psychological perspective the corona crisis is something experienced through the media and only rarely through personal experience. The self-amplifying effect in the so-called echo chambers has produced a kind of 'parallel reality' which, thanks to its continual fear mongering, has become the global irritant, manipulator and destabilising force in what were previously healthy social structures, something that would never have occurred without this media bluster. The threat posed by this globally connected world of the media is still insufficiently recognised.[120]

With the ability to transmit news and messages to every mobile phone in the world within a few minutes comes the possibility for awakening fear and manipulation on a scale that was never previously possible. And these opportunities are clearly being used more than we would like to believe. Already at the start of the 'pandemic' in April 2020 a secret strategy document from the German Home Office came into the public realm entitled 'How we bring covid-19 under control', in which guidelines were given under various headings for instilling the greatest amount of fear in the population. Fear of a million deaths, many critically ill patients dying at home 'struggling for air and suffocating' because overflowing hospitals had to turn them away. Children should also be feared because they pass on the infection so quickly. 'If they then infect their parents and one of them dies an agonising death at home and they think they might be to blame because, for example, they forgot to wash their hands after playing; this is the most dreadful thing a child could experience.'[121]

The authors of this secret paper were a 'group of experts' who almost with exception were economic professionals who it seems had been asked by the government to produce worst-case-scenarios to justify massive restrictions.[122] It is quite clear that the intention is not about providing factual information – the numerous nightmare scenarios make this abundantly clear – but about a conscious manipulation of behaviour by creating fear. The true motivation and key players behind such machinations remain largely hidden.

In the well-researched book, 'A State of Fear – how the British Government weaponised fear during the covid-19 pandemic',[123] the distinguished journalist Laura Dodsworth provides an insight into the fully fledged propaganda machine which the British Government used to drive the fear campaign in the context of the corona crisis. She shows in detail how with the help of behavioural psychology, specific emotionally loaded messages designed to increase the level of fear were released – the daily repetition of increasing infections and deaths, or the showing of shocking images of fearful, dying or dead people. Dodsworth gave numerous examples of how these images and statistics were being manipulated.

A key tactic is what the author describes as a 'Blitzkrieg of daily fear bombs' in the media, on posters in the streets, in shops and everywhere. Emotive, personalised messages were used – 'don't kill grandma', 'people will die', 'don't take Covid home with you this Christmas,' ' people will die if you break the rules', 'don't let a coffee cost a life'. We can all see what effect such 'fear bombs' can have on us and how they irritate our thinking, feeling and willing. There is a continuous threat of new deadly variants – the Italian, Brazilian, Kent, Indian, Nepalese… Each one is declared a huge threat, and if one disappears another new variant will feed the headlines. According to Dodsworth viruses are continuously mutating and there will always be new variants. Responding with glaring headlines each time, means there will always be an excuse to impose further repression and vaccination campaigns.[124]

Literature concerning what is really going on behind the official corona policies is readily available today, and it is shameful to observe how spinelessly and uncritically or perhaps even naively our politicians – and sadly many scientists, too – allow themselves to be taken in and misused by plutocratic megalomaniacs and their media enablers. Those in positions of responsibility must surely come to realise that something isn't right here and that it has very little to do with the health of the country's citizens but rather with a huge, multinational money-making scheme. In 2020 the turnover in mask sales was a massive 75 billion dollars,[125] 3.678 billion covid tests were sold (as of 22/2/2022)[126] each of which cost on average 75 Euros, amounting to a total of approx. 275 billion Euros. With regard to vaccines Pfizer alone can expect an income from its agreed delivery contracts around 33.5 billion dollars in 2021.[127] And it is quite clear that the global vaccination racket will be kept going using every tool available including what can only be described as the criminal plan to vaccinate children. It is only from an economic perspective that this story of a worldwide killer virus makes make any sense – continually new tests, new waves, new mutations, new vaccines. Humanity is being inoculated with fear in order to hide the truth. Covid-19 is the greatest cash cow in medical history.[128]

'They won't get out of this one in a hurry!', is a phrase heard ever more frequently in everyday conversations. The knowledge and state of awareness in the wider population is seemingly far broader and more differentiated than the repetitive mantra of fear propaganda that is being put out by the media. One of the most cunning ploys in terms of psychological technique is that of persuading large numbers of completely normal healthy human beings that there is a threat. Here again, age-old psychological patterns of guilt, such as that of the 'sinner', are activated and can only be redeemed by being 'good' and subjecting oneself unconditionally to the required rules.

The laws to be followed in this case, however, do not come from the guardians of a higher divine morality but from the dark chambers of a secret virology teaching that no human beings – not even the scientists themselves – are in a position to understand; their statements would otherwise not be so contradictory. That is why the 'ignorant masses' need strict guidance. 'Don't believe any rumours but only official pronouncements,' said Angela Merkel during a television address about the corona crisis on 18th March 2020.

Whoever wishes to invoke fear will hide the source of this fear in a mysterious, inaccessible cloak of darkness. We can after all only be afraid of what we don't know or understand. From the very beginning there was a very noticeable tendency to prevent a clear presentation of data. No random test analyses were carried out which is a pre-condition for any realistic epidemiology. A dubious non-validated PCR test was put in place without requiring any of the usual criteria to be met, and autopsies, which could have verified whether the cause of death was due to coronaviruses, were prohibited. The declaration by the WHO that everyone having a positive PCR test four weeks before their death should be registered as having died of Covid even though he may have died of cancer, a heart attack or even following an accident, is – to put it bluntly – utter nonsense. It merely demonstrates that the WHO, which receives 80% of its funding from major corporations, has become a puppet of the pharmaceutical industry.[129] 'Data on corona, a catastrophe' said Göran Kauermann, professor of statistics in Munich. Chaos and lack of transparency opens the door to arbitrariness – 'anything goes' – and hence also to manipulation.

Let us return now to the psychology of the apportioning of guilt in authoritarian systems. The power motive that once led the cleric to have his 'little sheep' confess to being sinners, make them fear eternal damnation and then set himself up as the one to rescue and bring them redemption, seems to be having a kind of renaissance today. This psychology currently manifests itself in the daily rituals of subjugation that occur when people with a more critical attitude are interviewed and then feel obliged to demonstrate their 'confession of faith' with: 'I am not an 'alternative thinker', antivaxxer, covid denier, conspiracy theorist etc'. They feel it necessary to pre-empt any accusation of the supposed guilt that hovers around. Some media professionals particularly like operating in this way and seek to draw out statements from their speaking partners which are then used to ridicule them publicly as 'antivaxxers'. An independent appraisal that does not conform to the mainstream view and its public backup is immediately considered suspect in these corona times – a symptom otherwise known only under totalitarian regimes.

The Austrian psychologist Alexander Meschnig in a recent and cleverly written essay 'The Covid Vaccine as Communion'[130], wrote about the 'redemption fantasies' in which the vaccine is touted as the only promise of salvation. The corollary is that covid deniers are then effectively 'God deniers'. By using the archaic struggle between good and evil – which of course never fails – this perfidious propaganda reanimates old religious patterns of behaviour. This is where the radicalisation of society originates with its increase in aggression and breakdown of relationships. According to Meschnig what we are facing is a battle between beliefs since all the figures used to justify the various measures have been refuted. The whole discourse about covid has therefore completely departed from reality.

There was the 'joyful message' from Bill Gates in his ten

minute address Easter 2020 as part of the main news bulletin that he would like to vaccinate the whole of mankind. And then at Christmas the first of those to be vaccinated were hailed with great pathos – finally salvation has come – in a celebration that never wanted to end.

Regression is the term used in psychoanalysis to describe a return to earlier stages in a personality's development when confronted with fear. This also applies to social-cultural processes. We must take great care in this present situation to ensure that the covid dictatorship does not result in societal regression and that our achievements in terms of a free, responsive and generally fair society are not crushed beneath the wheels of an antiquated, totalitarian dictatorship. These completely unnatural social distancing and hygiene ceremonies, especially the cringe-worthy elbow greetings and all the other comical and indeed inhuman prohibitions on direct contact not to mention the treating of unvaccinated people as outcasts, untouchables and criminals[131] seem quite absurd in modern times as does the treatment of people who think differently, the various forms of repression used and the lockdown measures that were so ruinous for many people. At times it seems as though we are developing backwards. That fact that all these shenanigans are completely unnecessary has been demonstrated in countries like Sweden.

The compulsory requirements are reminiscent of medieval cult slavery – there is even the morbid whiff of a mindset that bears resemblance to the inquisition. Just as at the end of the Middle Ages the spirit of the ancient world flowered once more during the Renaissance, so too are there negative examples of such rebirths. The increasing decadence and hence ever more war-like spirit dominating the church during the persecution of witches seems to be living again today in a new and heated up scenario of irrational fear. Although we have viruses today instead of witches, from a psychological perspective they are similar objects of fear. Both are catching and both spread harm. The 'promise of salvation' no longer comes from the house of God, but from the 'think tanks' of the vaccine industry. Just as in its time the church betrayed its spirituality and core Christian mission in favour of external power, so is science today in danger of squandering its true mission, the independent search for truth, to become the slave of alien interests and powers. In the Middle Ages the human quest for truth was answered by the revelation of faith. Since the Renaissance this role has been taken on to a certain extent by science, although at the present time its credibility is in danger of being lost. Perhaps corona is the crisis of a science that has become one dimensional?

'It will be a task of humanity to recognise the limitations of the great legacy that is our scientific culture, otherwise we will one day almost certainly annihilate ourselves.' Hans-Georg Gadamer[132]

A healthy human society thrives in the diversity of its individuals. It is precisely in the concurrence of unity and diversity that the art of democracy emerges. It is not a state of existence but a continuous process that lives through courage, commitment, presence of mind and the human capacity for dialogue. To this also belongs the emancipation from old psychological patterns woven out of fear and power.

Ecology and health

A genuine culture of health arises when we live in harmony with nature. Human health cannot be understood or maintained in future without taking the socio-ecological context into account.

The immunological stability of the human being depends to a large extent on the microbial cohabitants of our intestines. This internal ecosystem that we refer to as a microbiome and to which countless viruses, bacteria and other micro-organisms belong, is currently among the most studied fields of medicine. The knowledge coming to light, which in some areas is quite revolutionary, suggests a paradigm change is on its way in medical thinking. Research into the microbiome teaches us to take a *system-focused* approach through which we can gradually leave behind the one-dimensional causal logic of a mechanistic image of the human being to which we have been accustomed and learn to think in terms of broader interrelationships.

Each person's microbiome is very individually constituted and reflects the ups and downs of our physical and soul health as well as of our life situation and surroundings. Our microbiome is part of both the environment and our organism. Both systems observe the same ecological laws. In unhealthy surroundings our microbiome gets sick and with it the human being. This applies not only to biological but also to the psycho-social factors that affect the microbiome – what we call home reflects a mature harmony between the external and internal worlds on a biological as well as a soul level.

It grows increasingly clear: disease prevention is about nature protection. It is not about a struggle against micro-organisms but a new holistic awareness of ecology.[133] Viruses and bacteria are what could be called mediators between the micro and macro biosphere. Considerably more than 99 percent of these organisms have nothing to do with illness.

It is known today that the immune resistance of human beings to parasites and pathogens largely depends on the diversity and *individual* composition of our internal community of microbes. Our ego organisation influences this internal microsphere even as far as its composition and builds into it the most effective way of resisting the spread of pathological germs – also known as colonisation resistance. The more diverse, the more robust a system is both internally and externally. A healthy, natural meadow with a wide range of species is far more resistant to parasites than a vast over-fertilized field of maize. Parasites multiply far more quickly in monocultures than in mixed cultures. Infectious diseases are nothing but microbial monocultures that take hold and spread in unnatural and unhealthy habitats.

Biodiversity provides an important means for understanding the link between the micro-ecology of the human microbiome and the macro-biology of external nature. We can observe particularly in the western world not only a dramatic decline in the biodiversity of outer nature, for example a 70%-80% decline in the population of insects, but also among the micro-organisms both in agricultural soils and in the human digestive tract. A very simple rule can be applied to all these ecosystems – the greater the biodiversity the healthier and more robust is the system. Microbiomes, also in soils, are dynamic systems which, depending on external influences and changing environmental conditions, display an enormous degree of flexibility and capacity to adapt. It is via the micro-organisms to which viruses also belong, that nature's homoeostasis is stabilised, that is the fine and delicate state of balance that is health. If a healthy person travels to a faraway country where the water, climate and food is completely different, his microbiome will have to adapt, which often involves developing symptoms of diarrhoea. It can happen that certain kinds of intestinal bacteria which normally form 0.1% of the total flora, now multiply themselves due to the change in nutrition so that within 1 or 2 days they can make up 10% or 20% of the total. If the diversity of the intestinal microbiome is low then the range of options available to it for dealing with a change in conditions is also low – and this gives rise to illness.

The same thing applies to soils: Reduced microbial diversity increases the susceptibility for parasites; enzyme diversity and with it the metabolic repertoire, we could also say the 'livingness', declines. Soils under organic management have significantly more bacterial diversity and up to 80% more enzyme activity and therefore also a detoxifying function – greenhouse gases for example and especially laughing gas can be reduced quite significantly.[134]

The decline of microbial diversity in human beings, which today is primarily in industrial countries, has increased the predisposition for numerous illnesses. In the English speaking world (USA, Britain, Australia), for example, the number of children and young people with allergies is more than 30% while in Indonesia it is just 2%. Metabolic illnesses, obesity and psychological disorders are also on the rise. The more contact there is with different microbes during childhood the healthier will the developing immune system become. That is a scientific fact.[135] And high microbial diversity is what we gain primarily from our food which in turn comes from healthy soil.

The deeply embedded idea that viruses and bacteria are enemies is a phenomenon based less on biology than on psychology. It originated in the nineteenth century when infectious diseases were rampant and when scientists like Robert Koch and Louis Pasteur discovered certain microbes in the bodily secretions of those infected and declared them to be 'pathogens'. That was also very understandable because at that time there was no understanding for the complex nature of the human microbiome and its significance for health. Based on our modern understanding of micro-organisms we need to qualify the concept of pathogen. If a field is over-fertilised the diversity of meadow flowers will disappear and only dandelions will remain. We cannot say, however, that the dandelion is a pathogen; its mono-cultural presence is not the cause but a symptom of a disturbed system.

The human microbiome particularly in the intestines used to be known quite rightly as 'flora'. It has very much in common with the external plant world but with the one difference namely that the microbiome remains captive at a very early stage of development. We might call it the 'ur-biosphere within us'. Just as the macro-flora and especially indicator plants can tell us about soil properties and the qualities of the place, i.e. the state of the system, so too can the individual configuration of a person's micro-flora be an expression of their general state of health. And when certain types of microbes increase to excess, as occurs with an infectious illness, only rarely is exposure or direct infection the cause, rather it is the consequence of a systemic immunological weakness. Soil does not become sour because docks are growing there. On the contrary the sour soil favours the growth of docks, and it is very similar with the so-called pathogens. Viruses and bacteria, like the seeds of plants, are to be found everywhere and will only grow and thrive when the conditions are right.

The American microbiologist Elisabeth Costello from

Stanford University spoke of a paradigm change in medical research. For her, the principles developed by ecologists for exploring and understanding the earth as a whole can be used on a micro scale to investigate the intestinal microflora. In other words we should no longer look at viruses or micro-organisms in isolation but as a constituent part of a biological system. It is in this holistic perspective that the future lies. With this approach we can understand what infectious diseases and plagues are – essentially microbial mono-cultures which can only develop where there is imbalance or a problem of diversity created by ourselves.

Safeguarding the sphere of autonomy in human beings, animals and ecosystems creates a sustainable culture of health. We can also speak of an expanded ethical individualism which applies not only to single individuals but to the uniqueness of all cultural and biological systems and spheres. Wherever individual beings are able to show and express themselves – in nature *and* in culture – they are healthy. We can see this with every free-standing tree, animals in their natural habitats and in truly free human societies.

Where there is individual strength, no parasite can go – whether it be a biological or psychological phenomenon.

We may trust that our natural, ethical-moral feeling for nature has the same origin from which the healing forces of nature themselves arise.

Immunity against biological and spiritual infections, against what is parasitic and manipulative (alienation, fear, insinuation), whether it is biological or psychological, depends on the same basic forces of identity and authenticity – in effect on the individual or species-appropriate development of man and nature. Ecosystems such as a rainforest, coral reef, alpine valley or the heather moors of the Swabian Alps, have developed their unique character as ‘individuals’ over long periods of time.

Health and vitality, whether in the fields of ecology or culture, always arise out of diversity and the many-sided qualities of their constituent parts. Everything which contradicts this principle must be corrected with illness. Every attempt at uniformity, equalisation, state paternalism and standardisation, every monopoly and every superpower in the widest meaning of the word are in this sense all pathogenic factors. The tendency towards the colossal and imperial, the absolute and the totalitarian, to power of whatever colour, always collapses in the end because it goes against the natural law of diversity. *Monocultures are the true pathogens* – ecologically, economically, politically and culturally. The great problems of the world have always come about because of size, delusions of grandeur and the wish for ultimate control.[136]

Epilogue

What we are currently experiencing with this corona crisis is the threat of a new form of totalitarianism; the attempt at achieving under the guise of health provision, a standardised and uniform world. The image of viruses and bacteria as the enemy, is being misused to create fear and 'tyranny'[137] and along with this mistrust of 'wicked' nature, a growing sense of alienation between people.

The rejection of those who attempt to offer an explanation to the public in response to the very obvious confusion is a serious symptom of this. Likewise, the silence of those who, although seeing what is going on, do not want to entertain the risk of serious repression or social exclusion.

'To stand in the way of the pandemic machine would, in terms of one's own career, require suicidal idealism. Far better to row a safe course, howl with the wolves – or keep one's mouth shut.' (P. Schreyer) [138]

The concept of conspiracy theory is being so eagerly taken up by the media because they can use it as part of a refined psychological technique to discredit all dissenting voices. Obvious nonsense such as, 'we are being invaded by extra-terrestrials', is used to discredit justified criticism by lumping everything together as being highly suspect. The concept of conspiracy then loses its real significance – namely that secret discussions are taking place between certain interest groups to achieve criminal goals (which no doubt happens)

– and is misused to declare that all non-mainstream opinions are of psychopathic intent and therefore to be dismissed from any discussion. This concept encourages a certain laziness of thinking because it offers release from the burden of having to carry out one's own research or seek explanations while allowing those wishing to discredit other opinions to appear as enlightened realists. Diagnosing someone as a 'conspiracy theorist' makes it appear that we have a well-reasoned understanding of the situation in contrast to the demonstrating 'covidiots' – another concept which underlines the level of popularism to which our political vocabulary has already fallen. The purpose of politics is to create the conditions within which an open and transparent discourse can take place and which means that the rule of law should not determine but use all the means at its disposal to guarantee freedom of expression and independent thought.

The standard of information provided and the differentiation of views offered by our media has deteriorated to a shocking degree. Even among journalists the very things which do not belong to their profession, namely fear and conformity, rule the day. A constructive dialogue demands that the facts and sources of critical opinions are methodically investigated. Virtually none of this is currently happening. In order to have a comprehensive understanding of the situation we need to recognise the hugely problematic entanglement that exists between politics, industry and the media.[139] The growing fusion of these three realms has led to the formation of mighty power cartels which are increasingly undermining our democracy.

There is now sufficient literature criticising the pharmaceutical approach to fill half the libraries, and the authors are certainly no conspirators but competent professionals for whose courage, advice and concern we should be grateful. It is worthwhile reading some of these papers in order to understand the strategy that economic interests are seeking to implement in relation to the corona crisis.[140]

Politicians are seeing themselves as therapists, a role for which they are totally unsuited. Medical decisions such as for example whether to recommend vaccination must be given by doctors on an individual basis and not meted out by politicians or even corporations. Mandatory vaccination for covid-19 lacks any medical justification, has no scientific evidence to support it and is accompanied by incalculable risk. Mandatory vaccination by default is a real concern since those who are not vaccinated could be subjected to numerous forms of professional and social pressure until they give in and choose the lesser evil. In order to impose a worldwide annual vaccination programme – which is the economic motive driving this pandemic – further waves will be 'brought about' by increasing the numbers using this unreliable test. The precise number of false positives is not known, but even with declining numbers of infections they can still be used as an argument to show that the pandemic is still continuing.

The true, medically relevant data (infections that need treatment, the number of corona patients in hospital beds, utilisation of ventilators, mortality figures[141]) do not reveal any significant deviation from the long-term average. In summer 2020, the occupation of beds in intensive care units lay somewhat below 80% as they have done for many years (in Germany).[142] Following bed occupancy statistics for hospitals is, however, complex and can be very misleading. During 2020 there were 21 hospital closures in Germany. In addition, since summer 2020, the number of beds in intensive care wards has been *reduced* from 32,000 to 23,000, thus 9,000 taken out during corona time.[143] While personnel issues have contributed to this (e.g. lack of staff and reduced ratios in relationship to patients), even more important were funding stipulations: the state compensation payments for corona interventions are on the condition that bed occupancy in intensive care is at least 75%. At our clinic in Heidenheim, for instance, intensive care beds were reduced overnight from 22 to 16, resulting in a rise in bed occupancy from 72% to 100%.[144]

'There is a completely normal mortality rate in Germany,' said the virologist Hendrik Streeck in an interview with the columnist Wolfram Weimer in October 2020.[145] If the figures are higher in other countries, it will be due to causes other than the virus because that is the same everywhere.[146] Whether this normality is due to the lock down measures is not known since no definitive evidence is available – the various factors affecting mortality are much too complex. The often-quoted Sweden had a somewhat higher death rate – the average age of those who died was 84 – but in terms of the long-term average there was no significant deviation from the normal annual mortality which is subject to considerable seasonal variation in all countries. The seasonal flu outbreak of 2017 and the heat wave of 2018 are likely to have cost more lives than those lost in the corona year of 2020. Although 982,489 people, 48,000 more than the average for 2016-2019, died in Germany during 2020, this was to be expected even before the corona pandemic given the demographic data available - the population of Germany has been steadily increasing since 2012, with the number of people aged over 80 increasing by almost one million between 2016 and 2020, from 4,926,000 to 5,906,000. This means that the expected death figures which could be statistically expected, increased precisely as expected. As Göran Kauermann, biomathematist and President of the University of Munich stated: 'If an adjustment is made for the age effect, 2020 is not a noticeably conspicuous year'.[147]

As Hendrik Streeck goes on to point out, we should bring this over-dramatisation to a halt. The virus fear is frequently irrational and the tiniest of risks are being turned into major issues by the media and politicians. There is likely to be a further increase in the number of those testing positive – Streeck speaks of a permanent wave – as there is each year during the autumn and winter months. Ten times the number of new infections could then occur. We must finally rid ourselves of this crisis and panic mode, says Streeck.

This year we have the unprecedented situation that viruses found on human mucus membranes have been measured on a grand scale throughout the year right across the world. This has never happened before. We will only be able to judge the value of this data when a comparable amount of data, that is from other years, is available to compare. Only then will it be possible for these figures to be reliably assessed.

The widespread acceptance by the population of the restrictions placed on human contact (still) draws on the natural and deep-seated readiness to be helpful and on the self-evident need to protect our fellow human beings from harm. It becomes ever clearer, however, that *when everything is taken into account the damage caused by these measures will far exceed that of the virus!* This is something that everyone responsible needs to be personally clear about and account for.

The time is ripe once again for developing healthy common sense and greater trust instead of fear. We will have to live with coronaviruses and many other viruses in future, with infectious diseases and also with periods during the winter months when there is increased mortality. And we will need to become sufficiently sensitive to know whether such periods pose a genuinely serious threat requiring preventative measures or whether they are being instrumentalised for a globalised business model of society.

An important ethical question for the future will be whether we should value health protection above the inviolability of human dignity. Should not old people for instance, have the right to decide for themselves whether and to what extent they should be protected?

I consider it my duty as a doctor to present the situation here to the best of my knowledge and understanding. And everyone who does not make the effort to check things through carefully and seek explanations, shares responsibility for the drastic consequences of the global measures currently being taken.

Let us be open for a genuine and fair discussion. It is after all the very foundation of all healthy human culture.

Endnotes

Approximate English titles given in brackets for original German articles or publications.

1 Hardtmuth, T. 2019. 'Die Rolle der Viren in Evolution und Medizin – Versuch einer systemischen Perspektive' [The Role of Viruses in Evolution and Medicine – An Attempt at a Systemic Perspective]. In: *Jahrbuch für Goetheanismus 2019* [Yearbook for Goetheanism 2019]. Natural Science Section, Goetheanum, Dornach, Switzerland

2 Mölling, K. 2015. *Supermacht des Lebens – Reisen in die erstaunliche Welt der Viren* [Superpower of Life - Journeys into the amazing world of viruses]. München: C.H. Beck Verlag, pp. 106-107.

3 Gottschalk, M.G., Domschke K. 2018. 'Genetische Aspekte in der Ätiologie und Therapie von Angsterkrankungen' [Genetic aspects in the etiology and therapy of anxiety disorders]. In: Zwanzger P. (Ed.). *Angst: Medizin. Psychologie. Gesellschaft.* Berlin: Medizinisch Wissenschaftliche Verlagsgesellschaft.

4 Reche, I., D'Orta, G., Mladenov, N. et al. 2018. *Deposition rates of viruses and bacteria above the atmospheric boundary layer.* The ISME Journal (Int. Society for Microbial Ecology). 12: 1154–1162.

5 Hannigan, G.D., Meisel, J.S., Tyldsley, A.S. et al. 2015. *The Human Skin Double-Stranded DNA Virome: Topographical and Temporal Diversity, Genetic Enrichment, and Dynamic Associations with the Host Microbiome*. mBio 6 (5): e01578-15.

6 Mölling, K. 2015. op. cit., pp. 146-201.

7 Ryan, F. 2010. *Virolution – die Macht der Viren in der Evolution* [Virolution - the power of viruses in evolution]. Heidelberg:

Spektrum Akademischer Verlag, p. 60.

8 Mölling, K. 2015. Ibid, p. 40.

9 Kolata, G. 2002. *Influenza: Die Jagd nach dem Virus* [Influenza: The Hunt for the Virus]. Fischer Sachbücher, p. 11-47.

10 Villarreal, L.P. 2005. *Viruses and the Evolution of Life*. Washington: American Society for Microbiology, p. 128.

11 Witzany, G. 2009. *Biocommunication and Natural Genome Editing*, Springer, p. 134ff.

12 The studies into the reasoning behind mask wearing are contradictory. The supposed anti-viral protection is often not connected with viruses but with the reduced inhalation of dust which in turn reduces the risk of infection. Fine dust particles in the bronchial system reduce the immune functions. Prior to the corona crisis research studies found that masks offered no protection against viral infections. The supposed antiviral protection provided by masks is often linked not to the viruses but to the reduced inhalation of dust particles which in turn reduces the risk of infection.

13 Farber, C. 2020. *The Corona Simulation Machine: Why the inventor of the 'Corona Test' would have warned us not to use it to detect a virus*. https://uncoverdc.com/2020/04/07/was-the-covid-19-test-meant-to-detect-a-virus/, last accessed 14/04/2021

14 Mölling, K. 2015. *Supermacht des Lebens – Reisen in die erstaunliche Welt der Viren* [Superpower of Life - Travel into the amazing world of viruses]. München: C.H. Beck Verlag, p. 119-120.

15 Wichmann, D. 2020, *Autopsy Findings and Venous Thromboembolism in Patients With COVID-19*. In: Annals of Internal Medicine. https://www.acpjournals.org/doi/10.7326/M20-2003

16 As a comparison: If I am looking for the source of a certain quote, I can google the text and if the quote is stored somewhere on the internet the search engine will tell me where it comes from. Problems arise however if the quote is found in many different places that I know nothing of.

17 To do this the so-called primer is used to mark the beginning and end of the sequence being sought.

18 Kutter, S. 2014. Der Körper wird ständig von Viren angegriffen: Virologe Christian Drosten im Gespräch [The body is constantly attacked by viruses: an interview with virologist Christian Drosten]. https://tinyurl.com/Christian-Drosten-on-viruses, accessed 14/04/2021

19 Burger, K. 2016. Wie Viren unseren Darm beherrschen [How viruses rule our intestines]. https://www.spektrum.de/news/wie-viren-unseren-darm-beherrschen/1426006, accessed 14/04/2021

20 Malan, R. 2003. *Africa isn't dying of AIDS*, Spectator 2003. Quoted by Köhnlein, C., Engelbrecht T. 2020. *Viruswahn* [Virus-mania]. Lahnstein: emu-Verlag, p. 153 ff.

21 We use the concept of infection as it is used on a daily basis by the media even though it is not correct. The concept of infection is defined *as an invasion of the organism by a pathogen which causes a local or widespread condition of illness*. This is not the case with a mere positive test because with at least 80% of the positive tests there are no symptoms of illness in the organism. If references are made in the media to new infections it is a very misleading choice of words. The reference to 'those who have recovered' frequently used in the statistics, is also a misleading term since the majority of them were never ill.

22 Robert Koch Institut, 2020. *Bericht zur Optimierung der Laborkapazitäten zum direkten und indirekten Nachweis von SARS-CoV-2 im Rahmen der Steuerung von Maßnahmen* [Report into the optimisation of laboratory capacity for the direct and indirect verification of SARS COV 2 for providing guidance on measures to be taken]. 7.7.2020 (https://www.rki.de/DE/Content/InfAZ/N/Neuartiges_Coronavirus/Laborkapazitaeten.pdf?__blob=publicationFile)

23 Watson, J., Whiting, P.F., Brush, J.E. 2020. *Interpreting a covid-19 test result*. British Medical Journal, 369:m1808.

24 The number 1386 refers to the calculation example with a prevalence of 1000 infected persons per 100,000 inhabitants; the number 1399 refers to a more realistic prevalence of only one hundred per 100,000 inhabitants. In the whole Corona crisis, there has been a complete failure from the beginning to educate the public with solid, clean and well-understood data, so that we now have a kind of epidemiological 'ground fog' in which it is possible to manipulate statistics at will and easily.

25 Sönnichsen, Dr A., President Deutschen Netzwerks Evidenzbasierte Medizin e.V. [President of the German Network for Evidence-Based Medicine]. 2020. *COVID-19: Wo ist die Evidenz?* [Covid-19: where is the evidence?], https://tinyurl.com/COVID19--Wo-ist-die-Evidenz, Update 8/9/2020. Last accessed 14/04/2021.

26 Interview Sept. 2020 with Prof. Dr Harald Matthes, director of the hospital in Havelhöhe, Berlin in Info 3, '*Die Corona-Maßnahmen sind in dieser Pauschalität nicht mehr zu rechtfertigen*' [The corona measures can no longer be justified in this generalized manner]. https://tinyurl.com/info3-interview-covid-measures. Last accessed 14/04/2021.

27 Schlenger, R. 2020. *PCR-Tests auf SARS-CoV-2: Ergebnisse richtig interpretieren* [PCR tests for SARS-CoV-2: interpreting results correctly], https://tinyurl.com/PCR-richtig-interpretieren. In: Aerzteblatt.de online, and Deutsches Ärzteblatt print edition, 117, 24: 1194-1195, 12 June 2020.

28 Piatov, F. 2020. *Vier Kurven zur Gefahrenlage. Die Corona-Zahlen, die Sie wirklich kennen müssen* [Four curves on the danger situation. The Corona statistics you really need to know]. In: BILD Zeitung, 8/9/2020.

29 The virus burden among those who were HIV positive increased significantly following hurricane Katrina in south eastern USA as a result of heightened stress levels. https://www.intechopen.com/chapters/45003

30 Mandavilli, A. 2020. *Your Coronavirus Test Is Positive. Maybe It Shouldn't Be.* New York Times, 29/8/2020. https://www.nytimes.com/2020/08/29/health/coronavirus-testing.html

31 The PCR test is essentially a linear test which does not measure 'either/or' but 'how many'. When measuring blood pressure, I cannot say positive or negative but must relate the value to many other factors in order to assess it correctly.

32 Mandavilli, A. 2020. Op. cit.

33 In April 2021 the CDC published new laboratory testing guidelines that recommended reducing the RT-PCR-CT values to 28 cycles – with initial CDC guidance indicating this only be for fully vaccinated people who were tested for covid. The guidance was apparently only corrected months later. (https://childrenshealthdefense.org/defender/cdc-changes-rules-counting-breakthrough-cases/). The

lower CT value used meant that the number of those infected seemed to decline, which was then attributed to the vaccine. Only some labs appear to use the lower CT value; that labs do not publicise the CT values used makes meaningful comparisons of 'case' data virtually impossible.

34 *Revision of the Surveillance Case Definition for AIDS in Canada.* In: Canada Communicable Disease Report, Health and Welfare Canada Dez. 1993, p. 196.

35 Hardtmuth, T. 2017. *Medizin im Würgegriff des Profits* [Medicine in the stranglehold of profit]. Heidenheim: Amthorverlag.

36 Website for the Global Influenza Surveillance & Response System, https://www.gisaid.org/

37 See also the well-presented overview of the diversity of viruses in: Wodarg, G. 2021: *Falsche Pandemien. Argumente gegen die Herrschaft der Angst* [False pandemics: arguments against being ruled by fear]. München: Rubikon-Betriebsges.mbH, pp 107-137

38 https://www.youtube.com/watch?v=LBdkDYp9q6A

39 The argument that the increase in the number of cancer cases is connected with increasing life expectation is only partly true since there are increasing numbers of cases in children. Breast cancer cases which have doubled since 1970 are the most common cause of death amongst women aged between 30 and 60 in the western world. Three in ten women are younger than 55 when diagnosed.

40 Moustafa, A., Xie, C., Kirkness, E. et al. 2017. *The blood DNA virome in 8,000 humans.* Public Library of Science Pathogens, 2017; 13 (3). e1006292.

41 Dinse, G.E., Parks, C.G., Weinberg, C.R. et al. 2020. *Increasing Prevalence of Antinuclear Antibodies in the United States.* Arthritis & Rheumatology 2020; 72. pp. 1026-1035.

42 Blaser, M. J. 2017. *Antibiotika Overkill – So entstehen die modernen Seuchen* [Antibiotic overkill – this is how modern epidemics arise]. Freiburg: Herder Verlag.

43 Schneider, T. 2020. *Infektiologe an der Charité, Berlin.* In: Die Welt, 8/9/2020, p. 20.

44 Berufsverband Deutscher Internisten e.V. 2018. *Krebs erfolgreich mit Fieber behandeln* [Successfully treating cancer with a fever].

Internisten im Netz. https://www.internisten-im-netz.de/aktuelle-meldungen/aktuell/krebs-erfolgreich-mit-fieber-behandeln.html, 13/6/2018

45 Mawson A.R., Ray B.D., Bhuiyan A.R., Jacob B. 2017. *Pilot comparative study on the health of vaccinated and unvaccinated 6- to 12-year-old U.S. children.* Journal of Translational Science, 2017: DOI: 10.15761/JTS.1000186

46 Rosslenbroich, B. 2007. *Autonomiezunahme als Modus der Makroevolution* [Increasing autonomy as a goal of macroevolution]. Nümbrecht: Martina Galunder Verlag, p. 188-197.

47 Mölling, K. 2015. *Supermacht des Lebens – Reisen in die erstaunliche Welt der Viren* [Superpower of life - journey to the amazing world of viruses]. München: C.H. Beck Verlag. p. 219.

48 Nelde, A., Bilich, T., Heitmann, J.S. et al. 2020. *SARS-CoV-2 T-cell epitopes define heterologous and COVID-19-induced T-cell recognition.* Preprint at Research Square, https://doi.org/10.21203/rs.3.rs-35331/v1

49 Around 20 millions tests have been carried out in Germany since the beginning of the crisis, the average cost of laboratory analysis alone is about 50 Euros, for voluntary testing costs are somewhere between 90 and 240 Euros. https://praxistipps.chip.de/kosten-fuer-corona-test-wer-zahlt-eigentlich-was_119981

50 University Clinic of Tübingen 2018. *Neues Verfahren misst Immunantwort innerhalb von Minuten* [New method measures immune response within minutes]. https://www.medizin.uni-tuebingen.de/de/das-klinikum/pressemeldungen/66, 30/5/2018.

51 *Wo das Dogma beginnt, ist das Leben am Ende* [Where dogma begins is life at an end], brand eins magazine, https://www.brandeins.de/magazine/brand-eins-wirtschaftsmagazin/2002/selbststaendigkeit/wo-das-dogma-beginnt-ist-das-leben-am-ende

52 Compare Wilmanski, T., Diener, C., Rappaport, N. et al. 2021. *Gut microbiome pattern reflects healthy ageing and predicts survival in humans.* Nature Metabolism 2021; 3 (2). pp. 274–286. See also Zittlau, J. 2021. *Gut ist, was sich verändert* [Good is what changes], Die Welt, 6 April 2021, p. 20.

53 Holstein, T. 2019. Sport als Prävention: Fakten und Zahlen für das individuelle Maß an Bewegung [Sport as prevention: facts and

figures for the individual amount of exercise]. https://tinyurl.com/sport-als-praevention, Aerzteblatt.de.

54 Li, Q., Nakadai, A., Matsushima, H. et al. 2006. Phytoncides (wood essential oils) induce human natural killer cell activity. Immunopharmacology and Immunotoxicology 2006; 28 (2). pp. 319-333. https://pubmed.ncbi.nlm.nih.gov/16873099/

55 Holt-Lunstad, J., Smith, T.B., Layton, J.B. 2010. *Social relationships and mortality risk: a meta-analytic review*. PLoS Med 2010;7 (7): e1000316. doi: 10.1371/journal.pmed.1000316.

56 Taßler, J., Schmitt, J. 2020. *Beatmung bei Covid-19: Mehr Schaden als Nutzen?* [Ventilation for covid-19: More harm than good?]. https://www.tagesschau.de/investigativ/monitor/beatmung-101.html. In: Tagesshau, 30/04/2020. Last accessed 14/04/2021.

57 Ferner, R., Aronson, J.K. 2020. *Chloroquine and hydroxychloroquine in covid-19*. BMJ 369:m1432.

58 Fiolet, T., Guihur, A., Rebeaud, M.E. et al. 2020. *Effect of hydroxychloroquine with or without azithromycin on the mortality of coronavirus disease 2019 (COVID-19) patients: a systematic review and meta-analysis*. Clinical Microbiology and Infection, 26 August, 2020. DOI: https://doi.org/10.1016/j.cmi.2020.08.022

59 Schlimpert, V. 2020. *Auffallend viele Lungenembolien bei COVID-19-Intensivpatienten* [Noticeably high number of pulmonary embolisms in COVID-19 intensive care patients]. https://tinyurl.com/corona-lungenembolien1, Kardiologie.org, 27/4/2020, last accessed 14/04/2021

60 Püschel, K. et al. 2020. *Covid-19-Patienten sterben häufig an Thrombosen und Lungenembolien* [Covid-19 patients often die of thrombosis and pulmonary embolism]. https://tinyurl.com/corona-lungenembolien2, kma online, 11/05/2020. Last accessed 14/04/2021.

61 The studies on this are contradictory, with moderate usage positive effects are described, for example in Marseille by Didier Raoult. https://www.derstandard.de/story/2000116647564/der-wunderheiler-von-marseille, 9/04/2020.

62 Engelbrecht, T., Köhnlein, C.: *Die Medikamententragödie* [The medication tragedy]. https://www.rubikon.news/artikel/die-medikamenten-tragodie, Rubikon, 29.9.2020, last accessed

14/04/2021.

63 *Statement from the Chief Investigators of the Randomised Evaluation of COVid-19 thERapY (RECOVERY) Trial on hydroxychloroquine*, 5 June2020. https://www.recoverytrial.net/files/hcq-recovery-statement-050620-final-002.pdf

64 *USA liefern Brasilien Hydroxychloroquin* [USA supply Brazil with hydroxychloroquine], https://www.n-tv.de/politik/USA-liefern-Brasilien-Hydroxychloroquin-article21817027.html, NTV, 01/06/2020, last accessed 22/2/2022

65 Baars, C. et al. *Die Geschichte eines Hypes* [The story of a hype]. https://www.tagesschau.de/investigativ/ndr/chloroquin-bayer-101.html, Tagesshau, 15/06/2020. Last accessed 22/2/2022

66 Concorde Coordinating Committee. 1994. *Concorde: MRC/ANRS randomised double-blind controlled trial of immediate and deferred zidovudine in symptom-free HIV infection.* Vol. 343, Issue 8902, 9 April 1994, pp. 871-881. https://www.thelancet.com/journals/lancet/article/PIIS0140-6736(94)90006-X/fulltext. https://de.wikipedia.org/wiki/Zidovudin.

67 This subject is explored extensively by Köhnlein, C., Engelbrecht T. 2020. *Viruswahn* [Virus-mania]. Lahnstein: emu-Verlag, p. 93 ff.

68 Goethe, *Faust.* Translated by Anna Swanwick. Covent Garden: George Bell & Sons, 1879.

69 *COVID-19: WHO rät vom Einsatz von Remdesivir ab – Kortikosteroide nur bei schweren Verläufen* [COVID-19: WHO advises against the use of remdesivir - corticosteroids only in severe cases]. https://tinyurl.com/WHO-remdesivir, Aerzteblatt.de, 20/11/2020, last accessed 14/04/2021.

70 *Vom Katastrophenmodus der Politik zum risikostratifizierten Handeln* [From the disaster mode of politics to risk-assessed action]. Interview with Dr Harald Matthes, October 2020. https://tinyurl.com/erziehungskunst-Harald-Matthes. Erziehungskunst.

71 Soldner, G., Breitkreuz, T. 2020. *Covid-19.* Der Merkurstab 2020: 4. pp. 225-234. See also: https://medsektion-goetheanum.org/aktuelles/covid-19/

72 Büttner, C. 2020. *Informationen zu Erfahrungen mit Homöo-Prophylaxe (HP) bei Covid 19 in Kuba, China und Indien* [Information on Experiences with Homeopathic Prophylaxis

(HP) with Covid 19 in Cuba, China and India]. https://tinyurl.com/Ergebnisse-Homoeopathie; translation: https://tinyurl.com/Experiences-with-Homeopathic

73 Haseltine, W. 2020. *The Risks of Rushing a COVID-19 Vaccine*. Scientific American online, 22/06/2020. Editorial by the prestigious geneticist Prof. W. Haseltine from the Harvard Medical School. https://www.scientificamerican.com/article/the-risks-of-rushing-a-covid-19-vaccine/

74 Ibid.

75 Thrombosen nach COVID-19-Impfung: Theorie zur Pathogenese, Testung und Therapie [Thrombosis after COVID-19 vaccination: theory of pathogenesis, testing, and therapy], in online aerzteblatt.de, https://www.aerzteblatt.de/nachrichten/122232/Thrombosen-nach-COVID-19-Impfung-Theorie-zur-Pathogenese-Testung-und-Therapie, 19/3/21, last accessed 23/2/2022

76 Folegatti, P.D., Ewer, K.J., Aley, P.K. et al. 2020. *Safety and immunogeni of the ChAdOx1 nCoV-19 vaccine against SARS-CoV-2: a preliminary report of a phase 1/2, single-blind, randomised controlled trial.* The Lancet Aug. 2020; 396, pp. 467-478.

77 Heseltine, W. 2020. *The Risks of Rushing a COVID-19 Vaccine*. Scientific American online, 22/06/2020. https://www.scientificamerican.com/article/the-risks-of-rushing-a-covid-19-vaccine/

78 Cardozo, T., Veazey, R. 2020. *Informed consent disclosure to vaccine trial subjects of risk of COVID-19 vaccines worsening clinical disease*. The International Journal of Clinical Practice, 28 October 2020 https://doi.org/10.1111/ijcp.13795

79 Wie lässt sich die Impfbereitschaft in der Bevölkerung erhöhen? [How can the willingness to vaccinate be increased in the population?] https://www.hu-berlin.de/de/pr/nachrichten/mai-2021/nr-21510 , 10/5/21, last accessed 23/2/2022

80 COVID-19 Impfung für Kinder und Jugendliche? Vierzehn Argumente für einen rationalen Weg in Deutschland [COVID-19 vaccination for children and adolescents? Fourteen arguments for a rational path in Germany], https://www.researchgate.net/publication/351662151_COVID-19_Impfung_fur_Kinder_und_

Jugendliche_Vierzehn_Argumente_fur_einen_rationalen_Weg_in_Deutschland, ResearchGate, June 2021, last accessed 23/2/2022

81 Impfungen in Europa (Stand 05.04.21). https://www.politico.eu/article/coronavirusvaccination-europe-by-the-numbers/ (page subsequently removed)

82 CDC (2020) COVID-19 Vaccination. In: Cent. Dis. Control Prev. https://www.cdc.gov/coronavirus/2019-ncov/vaccines/safety/adverse-events.html. Accessed 8 May 2021 (page subsequently removed)

83 *Nobelpreisträger Luc Montagnier warnt vor dem mRNA-basierten Impfstoff gegen Covid* [Nobel laureate Luc Montagnier warns against mRNA-based covid vaccine], https://ruhrkultour.de/nobelpreistraeger-luc-montagnier-warnt-vor-dem-mrna-basierten-impfstoff-gegen-covid/, Ruhrkultour, 20/12/2020 interview. Last accessed 23/2/2022

84 Kustin T, Harel N, Finkel U, et al, 2021. *Evidence for increased breakthrough rates of SARS-CoV-2 variants of concern in BNT162b2 mRNA vaccinated individuals.* MedRxiv

85 *SARS-CoV-2 variants of concern and variants under investigation in England.* Technical Briefing 18, 2021. Public Health England, https://assets.publishing.service.gov.uk/government/uploads/system/uploads/attachment_data/file/1001358/Variants_of_Concern_VOC_Technical_Briefing_18.pdf, 9/7/2021

86 See also a commentary by scientific historian Prof. Harald Walach, *Unsere Impfstudie und unsere Kindermaskenstudie – Erläuterungen* [Our vaccination study and our child mask study - explanations], https://harald-walach.de/2021/07/19/impfstudie-kindermaskenstudie-erlauterungen/, 19/7/2021, last accessed 23/2/2022

87 Kowall, B., Standl, F., Oesterling, F. et al. 2021. *Excess mortality due to covid-19? A comparison of total mortality in 2020 with total mortality in 2016 to 2019 in Germany, Sweden and Spain.* Plos One 3/8/2021, https://doi.org/10.1371/journal.pone.0255540.

88 There are numerous reasons why this is different in other countries, but it cannot be due to the virus, which of course knows no national borders.

89 Voelkl, O. 2022. *Übersterblichkeit in Deutschland? Statistiken zu*

2022, 2021 und 2020 [Excess deaths in Germany? Statistics for 2022, 2021 and 2020], https://praxistipps.focus.de/uebersterblichkeit-in-deutschland-die-aktuelle-offizielle-statistik_128473, last accessed 23/2/2022

90 Matzenberger, M. 2021. *Weniger Covid-19-Opfer als letzten Herbst, aber höhere Übersterblichkeit* [Fewer Covid 19 victims than last autumn, but higher excess deaths], https://www.derstandard.de/story/2000131577990/weniger-covid-opfer-als-letzten-herbst-aber-hoehere-uebersterblichkeit, 2/12/2021, last accessed 23/2/2022

91 Deerberg, C. 2022. *Sieben wissenschaftliche Argumente gegen eine gesetzliche Impfpflicht* [Seven scientific arguments against mandatory vaccination], https://www.diekinderpraxis.de/2022/01/06/sieben-wissenschaftliche-argumente-gegen-eine-gesetzliche-impfpflicht/, 6/1/2022, last accessed 23/2/2022

92 Handelsblatt 2020. *Entwicklungsminister Müller: 'An den Folgen der Lockdowns werden weit mehr Menschen sterben als am Virus'* [Development Minister Müller: 'Far more people will die from the consequences of the lockdown than from the virus']. https://tinyurl.com/Entwicklungsminister-Muller, 22/9/2020

93 World Food Programme (WFP) 2020. *WFP Chief warns of hunger pandemic as COVID-19 spreads (Statement to UN Security Council).* https://www.wfp.org/news/wfp-chief-warns-hunger-pandemic-covid-19-spreads-statement-un-security-council, 21/4/2020, last accessed 22/4/2021.

94 Interview with Hendrik Streeck, Director of Virology at the University Clinic Bonn, *Corona-Pandemie: Virologe Hendrik Streeck will 'Virus nicht überdramatisieren'* [Corona pandemic: Virologist Hendrik Streeck does not want to 'overdramatize the virus']. https://web.de/magazine/news/coronavirus/virologe-hendrik-streeck-verbotspolitik-corona-pandemie-35144824, 8/10/2020, last accessed 22/4/2021.

95 Hardtmuth, T. 2017. *Medizin im Würgegriff des Profits* [Medicine in the stranglehold of profit]. Heidenheim: Amthor-Verlag. See also Light, D. et al. *Institutional Corruption of Pharmaceuticals and the Myth of Safe and Effective Drugs*, Journal of Law, Medicine and Ethics, Autumn 2013.

96 Global healthcare spending was around $ 8.5 trillion in 2018. This

is on average 10% of the worldwide gross domestic product of $ 84.9 trillion.

97 Mausfeld, R. 2019. Angst und Macht [Fear and power]. Frankfurt: Westendverlag.

98 Quoted from a book by Paul Schreyer with valuable explanatory contributions, *Chronik einer angekündigten Krise – wie ein Virus die Welt verändern konnte* [Chronicle of an announced crisis - how a virus could change the world]. Frankfurt: Westend-Verlag 2020, pp. 97-98.

99 Hollstein, T. 2019. *Sport als Prävention: Fakten und Zahlen für das individuelle Maß an Bewegung* [Sport as a preventative – facts and figures for the amount of individual movement]. Deutsches Ärzteblatt, 116: pp 35-36.

100 Schubert, C., Amberger, M. 2016. *Was uns krank macht, was uns heilt* [What makes us sick, what heals us]. Munderfing: Verlag Fischer & Gnann, pp. 70-73.

101 Weltbericht zum Artensterben: Das sind die erschreckenden Zahlen und Fakten [World report on species extinction: these are the terrifying facts and figures]. In Stern.de, https://www.stern.de/panorama/weltbericht-zum-artensterben--erschreckende-zahlen-und-fakten-in-der-uebersicht-8697780.html, 6/5/2019, last accessed 22/4/2021

102 In the six months up to September 2020, the net worth of the richest 643 Americans increased by 845 billion dollars. This is shown by the figures analysed in a new report by the Forbes Billionaire Rankings, the Americans for Tax Fairness (ATF) and the Institute of Policy Studies (IPS). The total net worth of the billionaires in the USA increased from 2.95 billion dollars to 3.8 billion dollars, an increase of 29% since 18th March. It is not only the pharmaceutical, digital and online trade corporations but also the financial sector which in the context of the investment programme has profited on a grand scale from the wave of new indebtedness caused by the Corona crisis. See: https://www.heise.de/tp/features/Um-845-Milliarden-US-Dollar-reicher-4906091.html (report 20/9/2020)

103 Fratzscher, M. 2021. Milliardäre sind die Pandemiegewinner [Billionaires are the pandemic winners], Zeit Online, https://www.zeit.de/wirtschaft/2021-05/vermoegenskonzentration-

corona-pandemie-ungleichheit-milliardaere-zunahme-reichtum-aktienmarkt, 20/5/2021, last accessed 23/2/2022.

104 Welt Hunger Hilfe. *Welthunger-Index* [World Hunger Index]. https://www.welthungerhilfe.de/hunger/welthunger-index/, 14/10/2020.

105 Ibid.

106 Oxfam Deutschland, *Neue Hunger-Epizentren durch Covid-19: Mehr Menschen könnten verhungern, als am Virus sterben* [New epicentres of hunger due to Covid-19: more people could starve than die from the virus]. https://tinyurl.com/neue-hunger-epizentren, 9/7/2020

107 Welt.de. 2018. *WHO: Weltweit jährlich rund sieben Millionen Tote durch Luftverschmutzung* [WHO: Worldwide around seven million die every year from air pollution]. https://tinyurl.com/Tote-durch-Luftverschmutzung, 2/5/2018, last accessed 23/2/2022.

108 Aerzteblatt.de. Drei Millionen Todesfälle jährlich durch Alkohol [Three million deaths every year from alcohol]. https://tinyurl.com/Alkolhol-Todesfaelle, 21/9/2018, last accessed 22/4/2021.

109 If the many billions of dollars paid out in this crisis had been invested in sustainable conservation and wisely conceived socio-ecological programmes it would have been a real blessing for the earth. See: Arvay, C. 2020. *Wir können es besser* [We can do better]. Köln: Quadriga-Verlag.

110 Wehling, E. 2017: *Politisches Framing. Wie eine Nation sich ihr Denken einredet – und daraus Politik macht* [Political framing: how a nation can talk itself into thinking a certain way – and make politics out of it]. Bonn: BPP.

111 *Kindermarketing für Lebensmittel* [Marketing of food to children], https://www.foodwatch.org/fileadmin/-DE/Themen/Kinderernaehrung/Marktstudie_Kinderlebensmittel_2021_foodwatch.pdf, 2021 study

112 Hamberger, B. 2017. *Diabetes tötet mehr Menschen als angenommen* [Diabetes kills more people than assumed], Gesundheitsstadt Berlin, https://www.gesundheitsstadt-berlin.de/diabetes-toetet-mehr-menschen-als-angenommen-11843, 9/11/2017, last accessed 23/2/2022

113 The Europe-wide EPIC study found that following just four basic

rules – no smoking, healthy diet, no obesity, regular exercise in fresh air – the risk of type 2 diabetes will be reduced by 93%.

114 Swiss historian Daniele Ganser gave an excellent public talk explaining the power of propaganda: https://www.youtube.com/watch?v=ooM3rrBoiBA (in German)

115 These images were less about multiple deaths than about a logistical problem caused the prohibition of burials. This was a fact that was not reported. In Italy the majority of those who die are normally buried. Now suddenly due to the hygiene regulations, everyone had to be cremated. This resulted in long queues forming in the mortuaries. At the request of the authorities the coffins were loaded on to lorries and brought to outlying crematoriums because the local centres were full to capacity. See: https://www.br.de/kultur/wieso-das-foto-des-militaerkonvois-in-bergamo-fuer-corona-steht-100.html

116 See also reference https://en.wikipedia.org/wiki/Nayirah_testimony

117 Müchler, G. 2002. *Medien und Gewalt* [Media and violence], in Die Politische Meinung, No. 391, June 2002, https://www.kas.de/c/document_library/get_file?uuid=c2065875-2886-2c0e-6b07-21a897ce961c&groupId=252038

118 *Mehr Jugendliche mit depressiven Symptomen* [More youth with symptoms of depression], https://www.tagesschau.de/inland/gesellschaft/corona-depressionen-jugendliche-101.html, Tagesschau, 28/7/2021, last accessed 23/2/2022.

119 Südwestpresse newspaper, 18.8.2021

120 Just two small examples: When the football star Christiano Ronaldo declined coca cola in favour of mineral water during a television interview, Coca Cola's shares fell. That it is possible to manipulate the stock market for profit by engineering such effects is obvious. Pfizer's chief executive Albert Bourla, had a long term plan to sell a large proportion of his shares and decided to do so on the very day when the apparent effectiveness of the Pfizer vaccine was publicised across the globe and drove up the value of Pfizer shares. He then made a profit of many millions of dollars on one day. (https://www.businessinsider.de/wirtschaft/finanzen/pfizer-chef-verkauft-60-prozent-der-aktien-am-tag-der-corona-impfstoff-bekanntgabe/)

121 *Wie wir COVID-19 unter Kontrolle bedommen – Strategiepapier des Bundesinnenministeriums* [How we bring covid-19 under control – Strategy paper of the Federal Ministry of the Interior], https://fragdenstaat.de/dokumente/4123-wie-wir-covid-19-unter-kontrolle-bekommen/, last accessed 23/2/2022

122 Dosideit, A and Nabert, A. 2021, *Wenn der Staatssekretär Wissenschaftler zu „maximaler Kollaboration" aufruft* [When the State Secretary calls on scientists to "maximise collaboration"], https://www.welt.de/politik/deutschland/plus225868061/Corona-Politik-Wie-das-Innenministerium-Wissenschaftler-einspannte.html, Welt online, 8/2/2021, last accessed 23/2/2022

123 Dodsworth, L. 2021. *A State of Fear: How the UK Government Weaponised Fear During the Covid-19 Pandemic,* London: Pinter & Martin, 2021, 320 pp, ISBN 978-1-78066-720-1

124 Quoted from a review by Richard Brinton, Stroud, GB. https://ahpb.org/index.php/nl-2021-t7-16-a-state-of-fear-review-2/

125 Das Geschäft mit der Maske [The business with the masks], https://www.deutsche-bank.de/ms/results-finanzwissen-fuer-unternehmen/maerkte/03-2021-das-geschaeft-mit-der-maske.html, March 2021, last accessed 23/2/2022

126 Anzahl durchgeführter Tests für das Coronavirus (COVID-19) in ausgewählten Ländern [Number of tests performed for coronavirus (COVID-19) in selected countries], https://de.statista.com/statistik/daten/studie/1105095/umfrage/anzahl-durchgefuehrter-tests-fuer-das-coronavirus-nach-laendern/, last accessed 23/2/2022

127 https://www.manager-magazin.de/unternehmen/pharma/pfizer-covid-19-impfstoff-spuelt-34-milliarden-dollar-in-die-kasse-a-49c8253c-b758-4c39-aed4-4d3b2322e601. Latest February 2022 news release: *Pfizer reports nearly $37 billion in COVID-19 vaccine sales in 2021,* Washington Examiner, https://www.washingtonexaminer.com/policy/healthcare/pfizer-reports-nearly-37-billion-in-covid-19-vaccine-sales-in-2021, report 8/2/2022, last accessed 23/2/2022.

128 Psycho-neuroimmunologist Prof. Dr. Christian Schubert quoted in an interview with Alexander Gloog, *'Dummheit und Profitgier – Impfen bei Angst'* [Stupidity and greed – Vaccination out of fear], https://qs24.tv/2021/04/06/20-jahre-kuerzer-leben/

129 *Die Pharma-Lobby kontrolliert die Weltgesundheits-Organisation*

[The Pharma lobby controls the WHO], https://deutsche-wirtschafts-nachrichten.de/503554/Die-Pharma-Lobby-kontrolliert-die-Weltgesundheits-Organisation, 18/4/2020, last accessed 23/2/2022.

130 Meschnig, A. *Die Corona-Impfung als Kommunion* [The Corona vaccine as communion], https://www.achgut.com/artikel/die_spritze_als_kommunion, 13/7/2021, last accessed 25/2/2022.

131 The appalling brutality of the police at the demonstration in Berlin on August 1st 2021 led to the UN special correspondent for torture asking the Swiss law scientist Nils Melzer to investigate and called on the German government to explain itself.

132 Gadamer, H.G., Quote from an interview with Rüdiger Safranski. https://kzhome.info/crone/05WQsZiKZHCQlYU/hans-georg-gadamer-gespr-ch-mit-r-diger-safranski, last accessed 25/2/2022.

133 Hardtmuth, T. 2020. 'Das Corona Syndrom – warum die Angst gefährlicher ist als das Virus' [Corona Syndrome - why fear is more dangerous than the virus]. In: Eisenstein, C, Hardtmuth, T., Hueck, Chr., Neider, A. 2020 *Corona und die Überwindung der Getrenntheit* [Corona and overcoming separation]. Akanthos Akademie Edition Zeitfragen, p. 11-48.

134 Skinner, C., Gattinger, A., Krauss, M. et al. 2019. *The impact of long-term organic farming on soil-derived greenhouse gas emissions*. Scientific Reports 2019; 9 (1). Artikelnr. 1702.

135 Having air filtration systems in classrooms has no scientific basis. It may be one of the lucrative pandemic business models but it has nothing to do with health. Quite the contrary we 'benumb' the immune system of children with it. Coming up with such a grotesque idea at all is a symptom of the over blown paranoia of fear we are surrounded with today.

136 At this point it is worth remembering the economist and philosopher Leopold Kohr (1909-1994) whose life work, *Die Kritik der Größe* [Critique of grandeur], has great relevance for today's situation.

137 In a lecture given in 1909 Rudolf Steiner made some prophetic comments: 'What for instance would mankind be facing if fear of bacilli were to be exploited and legally enforced rules were created to fight these bacilli. (….) All this cannot be controlled but it would lead to impossible conditions, to unbearable tyranny.' Quoted from Claudius Weise, *Auch eine Sezession* [Also a sezession]. Die Drei

10/2020, p. 61.

138 Schreyer, P. 2020. *Chronik einer angekündigten Krise – wie ein Virus die Welt verändern konnte* [Chronicle of an announced crisis - how a virus could change the world]. Frankfurt: Westend-Verlag, p. 142.

139 An example is given of the German minister of health, Jens Spahn, who before taking up his ministerial role had been a lobbyist for the medical-pharmaceutical firm which he himself had founded and which is represented at numerous elite gatherings of global industry and finance such as the Bilderberg conferences. His partner is the chief lobbyist for Hubert Burda Media KG, one of the largest media organisations in Germany (Bunte, Focus, Freundin and many more). These journals have considerable influence on public opinion and they are unlikely to have any critical comments about Jens Spahn or Corona policies. To confer on a former pharmaceutical lobbyist the sole power to manage a health crisis that will prove extremely lucrative for the pharmaceutical concern without any parliamentary scrutiny, must inevitably lead to mistrust and scepticism in a democracy.

140 The following are named as examples: Köhnlein, C., Engelbrecht T. 2020. *Viruswahn* [Virus-mania]. Lahnstein: emu-Verlag; Schreyer P. 2020. *Chronik einer angekündigten Krise – wie ein Virus die Welt verändern konnte* [Chronicle of an announced crisis - how a virus could change the world]. Frankfurt: Westend-Verlag. Reiss, K., Bhakdi, S. 2020. *Corona, false alarm? Facts and Figures.* Chelsea Green Publishing Co.

141 Statista. *Anzahl der Sterbefälle in Deutschland von März 2019 bis März 2021* [Number of deaths in Germany from March 2019 to March 2021]. https://tinyurl.com/sterbefaelle-in-deutschland

142 Verfügbare und belegte intensivmedizinische Betten in Deutschland [Available and occupied intensive care beds in Germany], https://de.statista.com/statistik/daten/studie/1109137/umfrage/verfuegbare-und-belegte-intensivmedizinische-betten-in-deutschland/, last accessed 21/4/2021.

143 Merkur.de. *Corona: 9.000 Intensivbetten weniger als noch 2020: Warum sie häufiger 'gesperrt' werden, ist alarmierend* [Corona: 9,000 fewer intensive care beds than in 2020: Why they are being 'blocked' more often is alarming], https://tinyurl.com/9000-Intensivbetten-weniger, 9/4/2021, last accessed 25/2/2022]

144 That hospitals are 'overwhelmed', which we hear almost every day in the news, is thus less of a Corona problem than a political problem. In Italy, EU austerity measures have led to even more radical cuts in beds, which, as expected, led to dramatic bottlenecks in intensive care wards.

145 Hendrik Streeck, Director of Virology at the University Clinic Bonn, *Corona-Pandemie: Virologe Hendrik Streeck will 'Virus nicht überdramatisieren'* [Corona pandemic: Virologist Hendrik Streeck does not want to 'overdramatize the virus']. https://web.de/magazine/news/coronavirus/virologe-hendrik-streeck-verbotspolitik-corona-pandemie-35144824, 8/10/2020, last accessed 22/4/2021.

146 De.Statista.com. *Verfügbare und belegte intensivmedizinische Betten in Deutschland* [Available and occupied intensive care beds in Germany], https://tinyurl.com/tn7hne2b, last accessed 21/4/2021

147 *Focus online. Massive Kritik an Pandemie-Behörde: Statistiker holt zur RKI-Schelte aus: Corona-Daten 'eine einzige Katastrophe'* [Massive criticism of the pandemic authority: Statistician scolds RKI (Robert Koch Institute): Corona data 'an absolute catastrophe']. https://tinyurl.com/kritik-an-pandemie-behoerde, 31/1/2021, last accessed 22/4/2021.

About the Author

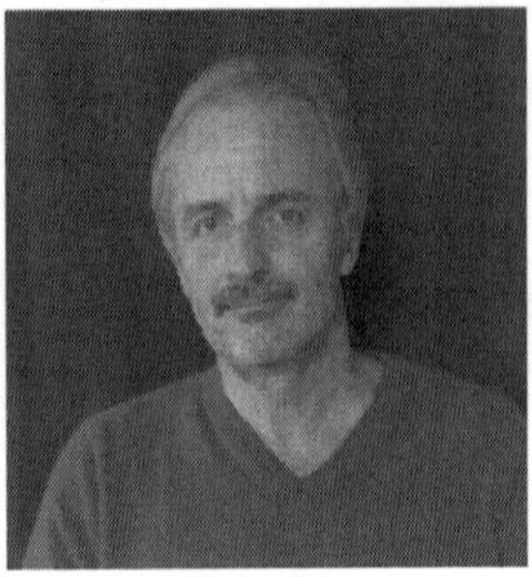

Dr. med. Thomas Hardtmuth is a specialist in general surgery/ thoracic surgery, freelance author, and long-time lecturer in health sciences and social medicine at the Baden-Württemberg University of Applied Sciences. He studied medicine at the TU and LMU Munich. He has been working as a doctor in various clinics in southern Germany since 1985, most recently as senior physician for general surgery and thoracic surgery at the Heidenheim Clinic. Virology and the role of viruses in nature and evolution is an area of research specialisation.

Dr Hardtmuth has published numerous articles and books, most in German. These include: (approximate English translation of German titles in brackets)

- *Das verborgene Ich – Aspekte zum Verständnis der Krebskrankheit* [The hidden self - aspects for understanding cancer], Amthorverlag, Heidenheim 2003

- *In der Dämmerung des Lebendigen – Hintergründe zu Demenz, Depression und Krebs* [In the twilight of life – backgrounds to dementia, depression and cancer], Amthorverlag, Heidenheim 2011

- *Medizin im Würgegriff des Profits – die Gefährdung der Heilkunst durch die Gesetze der Ökonomie* [Medicine in the stranglehold of profit - the danger to the art of healing through laws of economics], Amthorverlag, Heidenheim 2017

- *Das Mikrobiom des Menschen. Die Bedeutung der Mikroorganismen und Viren in Medizin, Evolution und Ökologie – Wege zu einer systemischen Perspektive* [The human microbiome. The importance of microorganisms and viruses in medicine, evolution and ecology – ways to a systemic perspective]. Salumed-Verlag, Berlin. June 2021.

Other books published by InterActions

https://interactions360.org

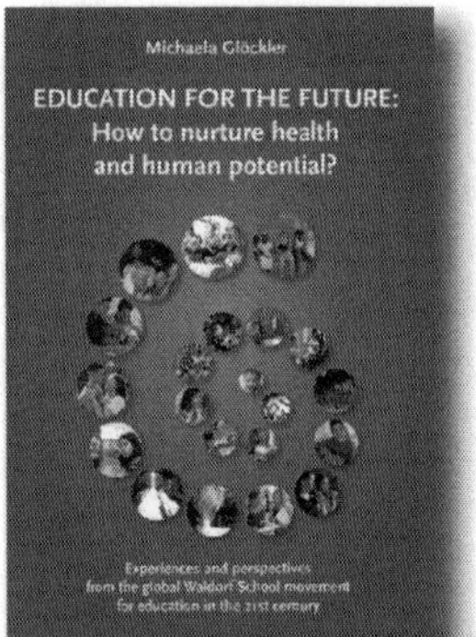

EDUCATION FOR THE FUTURE:

How to nurture health and human potential

by Michaela Glöckler, MD

2020. ISBN 978-0-9528364-3-8
UK price £19.99
Pb. 248 pp, colour illustrations.

Education for the Future is a plea for radically aligning upbringing and education with what is needed for the healthy development and well-being of children and adolescents. A unique contribution of Dr Glöckler is a year-by-year examination of human biological development and how this relates to soul-spiritual development, which in turn has a direct bearing on the needs of the child within upbringing and education. A treasure chest of information and insights for educators, parents, carers and therapists.

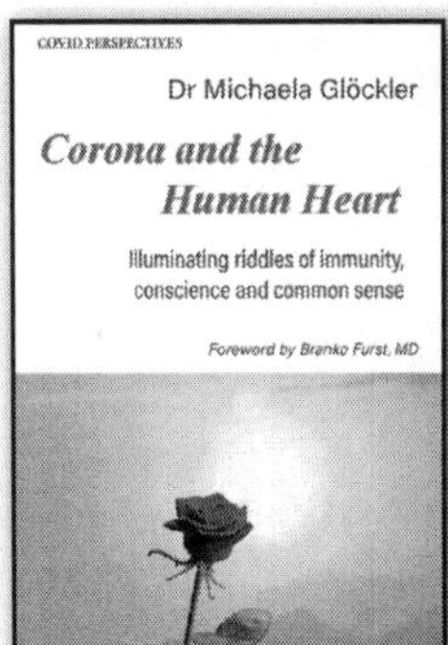

CORONA AND THE HUMAN HEART

Illuminating riddles of immunity, conscience and common sense

by Michaela Glöckler, MD

Foreword by Branko Furst, MD

2021. ISBN 978-0-9528364-5-2. Pb. 96 pp
colour and B&W illustrations, UK £7.95

New inspiring research on the significant role of the heart in the development of the immune system and the importance this understanding has for health and for the Covid crisis. The author leads us on a path showing how by strengthening our inner spiritual self – our inner sun – we will be strengthening our health and immunity, as well as illuminating riddles of conscience and common sense.

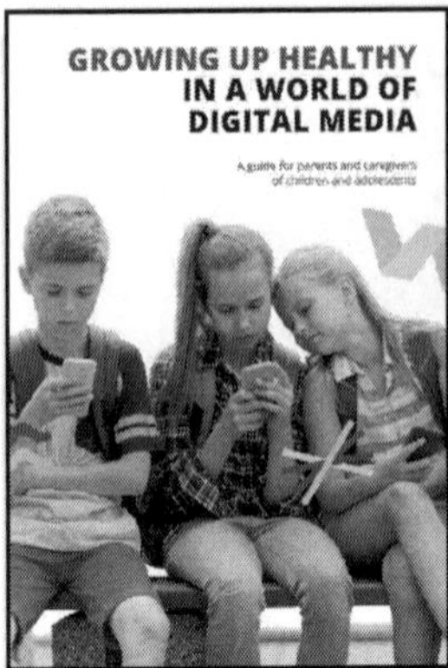

GROWING UP HEALTHY IN A WORLD OF DIGITAL MEDIA

Written by specialists from 15 organisations concerned with childhood development. Introduction by Dr Michaela Glöckler, Pediatrician

2019. ISBN 978-0-9528364-1-4
Sewn pb. 160 pp, colour illustrations and photos. UK £10

With increased screen use from the epidemic lockdowns, this new guide is more relevant than ever. It explains essential child development considerations for an age appropriate use of digital media. The risks from inappropriate use of digital media are considerable. This book offers practical advice to parents and teachers, divided according to children's age groups. *An essential guide.*

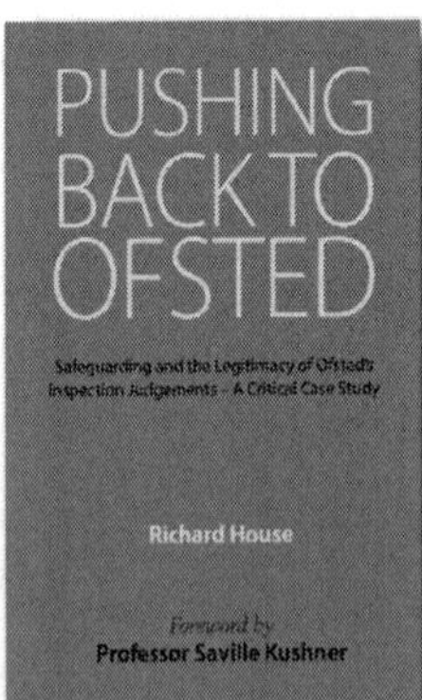

PUSHING BACK TO OFSTED

Safeguarding and the Legitimacy of Ofsted's Inspection Judgements – A Critical Case Study

by Richard House
Foreword by Prof. Saville Kushner

2020. ISBN 978-0-9528364-2-1
Pb. 128 pp Pb. UK £10.99

'...This analysis of one significant but not unique example of the problems that can arise with school inspections is an uncomfortable but necessary challenge to current educational orthodoxies.'
Dr. Rowan Williams, former Archbishop of Canterbury

Dr House sets out in relentless detail the shortcomings and prejudices of the Ofsted report for a UK Waldorf school as an example for how a state's one-size-fits-all approach can perpetuate a kind of violence on educational creativity and freedoms. A helpful study for schools facing intense state scrutiny and judgement.

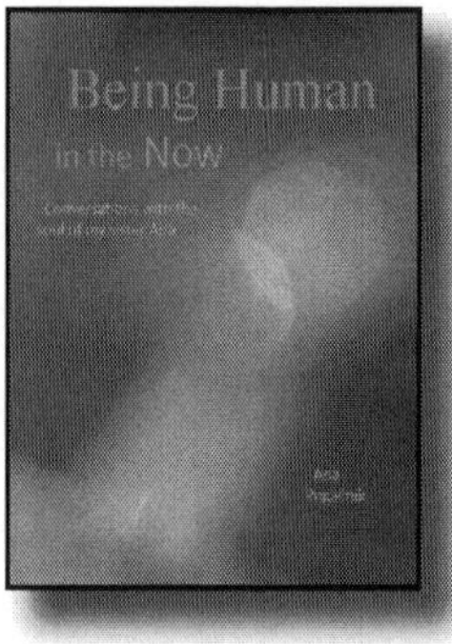

BEING HUMAN IN THE NOW: Conversations with the soul of my sister Ajra

by Ana Pogacnik

2022. ISBN 978-9528364-6-9
Pb 120 pp. With illustrations. UK £12

Ten years after her death, the author takes up conversations with the soul of her parted sister, revealing profound insights into challenges humanity is facing. The themes covered are direct, detailed and breathtakingly lively and highly topical, from the increasing difficulties souls have in crossing the threshold, to current topics affecting this including suicides, medications and the dangers of the new mRNA vaccinations with their ability to penetrate the 'divine script' of our body. Inspiring are the descriptions of the deep significance of love as a source of strength, and of the spiritually radiating living being we know as earth which we can learn to interact with. In all of this the message is: the departed souls are there to help us if we have the courage and fortitude to open ourselves to them.

Upcoming InterActions publications

(Provisional titles and details - see website for updates)

BEYOND BIO-MEDICINE

Towards a new paradigm for health and well-being

In this extended interview-dialogue, **Dr Thomas Hardtmuth** and **Richard House Ph.D.** dive deeply into the very foundations of human well-being, exhaustively detailing what is wrong philosophically and clinically with the current prevailing biomedical paradigm of health and disease; how these shortcomings have been highlighted in the course of the Covid crisis; and what changes need to occur for the radical re-founding of a genuinely holistic understanding of health, illness and healing to occur. **Publication spring 2022.**

LIMITS TO MEDICAL SCIENCE:

'Revolutionary' Conversations.

Interviews with medical professionals, philosophers, psychologists and researchers. **Publication in 2022.**